MW00344583

Second
UPDATED
Edition

Curbside Consultation in Cataract Surgery

49 Clinical Questions

CURBSIDE CONSULTATION IN OPHTHALMOLOGY
SERIES

SERIES EDITOR, DAVID F. CHANG, MD

Second
UPDATED
Edition

Curbside Consultation in Cataract Surgery

49 Clinical Questions

Editor
Terry Kim, MD
Professor of Ophthalmology
Duke University School of Medicine
Cornea and Refractive Surgery Service
Duke University Eye Center
Durham, North Carolina

Associate Editors
Derek W. DelMonte, MD
Assistant Professor of Ophthalmology
Duke University School of Medicine
Cornea and Refractive Surgery Service
Duke University Eye Center
Durham, North Carolina

Preeya K. Gupta, MD
Assistant Professor of Ophthalmology
Duke University School of Medicine
Cornea and Refractive Surgery Service
Duke University Eye Center
Durham, North Carolina

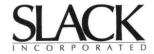

SLACK
INCORPORATED

www.Healio.com/books

ISBN: 978-1-61711-088-7

Copyright © 2014 by SLACK Incorporated

All rights reserved. No part of this book may be reproduced, stored in a retrieval system or transmitted in any form or by any means, electronic, mechanical, photocopying, recording or otherwise, without written permission from the publisher, except for brief quotations embodied in critical articles and reviews.

The procedures and practices described in this publication should be implemented in a manner consistent with the professional standards set for the circumstances that apply in each specific situation. Every effort has been made to confirm the accuracy of the information presented and to correctly relate generally accepted practices. The authors, editors, and publisher cannot accept responsibility for errors or exclusions or for the outcome of the material presented herein. There is no expressed or implied warranty of this book or information imparted by it. Care has been taken to ensure that drug selection and dosages are in accordance with currently accepted/recommended practice. Off-label uses of drugs may be discussed. Due to continuing research, changes in government policy and regulations, and various effects of drug reactions and interactions, it is recommended that the reader carefully review all materials and literature provided for each drug, especially those that are new or not frequently used. Some drugs or devices in this publication have clearance for use in a restricted research setting by the US Food and Drug and Administration or FDA. Each professional should determine the FDA status of any drug or device prior to use in his or her practice.

Any review or mention of specific companies or products is not intended as an endorsement by the author or publisher.

SLACK Incorporated uses a review process to evaluate submitted material. Prior to publication, educators or clinicians provide important feedback on the content that we publish. We welcome feedback on this work.

Published by: SLACK Incorporated
                       6900 Grove Road
                       Thorofare, NJ 08086 USA
                       Telephone: 856-848-1000
                       Fax: 856-848-6091
                       www.Healio.com/books

Contact SLACK Incorporated for more information about other books in this field or about the availability of our books from distributors outside the United States.

Library of Congress Cataloging-in-Publication Data
Curbside consultation in cataract surgery : 49 clinical questions / [edited by] Terry Kim. -- Second edition.
  p. ; cm.
Includes bibliographical references and index.
ISBN 978-1-61711-088-7 (paperback : alk. paper)
I. Kim, Terry, editor of compilation.
[DNLM: 1. Cataract Extraction--methods. WW 260]
RE451
617.7'42059--dc23
2013033369

For permission to reprint material in another publication, contact SLACK Incorporated. Authorization to photocopy items for internal, personal, or academic use is granted by SLACK Incorporated provided that the appropriate fee is paid directly to Copyright Clearance Center. Prior to photocopying items, please contact the Copyright Clearance Center at 222 Rosewood Drive, Danvers, MA 01923 USA; phone: 978-750-8400; website: www.copyright.com; email: info@copyright.com

Printed in the United States of America.

Last digit is print number: 10 9 8 7 6 5 4 3 2 1

Dedication

To my wife, Ellie, and my children, Ashley and Kayley, for their never-ending love, support, and understanding.

To my parents, Kyung Hwae and Hyun Sim Kim, for raising, educating, supporting, and taking care of me.

To all my resident, fellow, and medical student trainees, for constantly stimulating my mind, inspiring me to be a better teacher, and keeping me young.

To all my faculty and colleagues at Duke University, Duke University School of Medicine, and Duke University Eye Center, who have been a pleasure and privilege to practice, research, and collaborate with, and who have supported my career.

To all my mentors, teachers, and colleagues, for their advice, guidance, encouragement, and friendship throughout my career. I would particularly like to thank the following for their impact on my career: Drs. Thomas Aaberg, Amar Agarwal, Ike Ahmed, Steve Arshinoff, Rosa Braga-Mele, Geoffrey Broocker, Reay Brown, Francesco Carones, David Chang, Y. Ralph Chu, Robert Cionni, Elisabeth Cohen, Garry Condon, Alan Crandall, Uday Devgan, Eric Donnenfeld, Henry Edelhauser, David Epstein, Howard Fine, James Gills, Sadeer Hannush, David Hardten, Bonnie Henderson, Warren Hill, Richard Hoffman, Jack Holladay, Edward Holland, John Hovanesian, Choun-Ki Joo, Eung Kweon Kim, Jae Ho Kim, Douglas Koch, Jay Krachmer, Peter Laibson, Stephen Lane, Richard Lewis, Richard Lindstrom, Jodi Luchs, Robert Machemer, Richard Mackool, Francis Mah, Parag Majmudar, Nick Mamalis, Mark Mannis, Samuel Masket, Kevin Miller, Louis "Skip" Nichamin, Thomas Oetting, Robert Osher, Richard Packard, David Palay, Frank Price, Irv Raber, Michael Raizman, Christopher Rapuano, David Ritterband, Richard Rodman, Thomas Samuelson, Vincenzo Sarnicola, Aryan Shayegani, John Sheppard, Allan Slomovic, Kerry Solomon, Walter Stark, Roger Steinert, Doyle Stulting, Hungwon Tchah, Mark Terry, Richard Tipperman, William Trattler, David Vroman, Keith Walter, George Waring III, Won Ryang Wee, and Sonia Yoo.

Terry Kim, MD

To my father, for his inspiration; to my chief resident, Tarra Millender, for her patience and education; and to my many mentors, especially Richard Forster, for their never-ending commitment to the next generation of ophthalmologists.

Derek W. DelMonte, MD

I dedicate this book to my family; my husband, Rajan; and my daughters, Meera and Siyona, for their love, support, and patience; to my parents, for being amazing role models and for giving never-ending love and encouragement; and to all of my mentors who have taught me that there is always more to learn, more to see, and barriers to cross.

Preeya K. Gupta, MD

Contents

Acknowledgments

We are fortunate to have so many bright, talented, creative, and passionate leaders in our field who take altruism at heart and devote their free time to educate us through meetings, conferences, symposia, peer-reviewed articles, trade journals, and other media. We would like to take this opportunity to thank these leaders who have taken extra efforts to contribute to this unique textbook on cataract surgery.

First and foremost, we would like to acknowledge Dr. David F. Chang for his inspiration and initiative for coming up with yet another well-received and popular format for this book, as well as the *Curbside Consultation* series as a whole. His boundless energy and lead-by-example style has encouraged all of us to work harder to educate those who are in training, are abroad, and are less fortunate than us in terms of their resources for learning.

Second, we thank all of our contributing authors for taking time out of their busy schedules to share their knowledge and wisdom. They were all sought out for their expertise in their respective areas in cataract surgery, and they all answered their questions in their own personal style and in a timely fashion, just as they would if they were asked the question in person, on the phone, or via email. We are indebted to our cataract experts, for it is their reputation and expertise that makes this book such a valuable and special resource.

Third, we would also like to recognize the numerous residents and clinicians in both private practice and academic environments that assisted us in reviewing and critiquing the *Curbside* questions as well as the responses: Rosa Braga-Mele, Geoffrey Broocker, Bonnie Henderson, Tim Johnson, Ed Kim, Donna Lee, Scott Lee, Jeff Maassen, Hunter Newsom, Erin O'Malley, Luis Omphroy, Steve Sauer, Pulin Shah, Andrew Sorenson, George Yang, and Sonia Yoo.

In addition, we are extremely grateful to John Bond and his wonderful and resourceful team at SLACK Incorporated's Health Care Books and Journals Division. Their professionalism, guidance, and dedication to this project helped make this book a reality and a success. We would specifically like to thank the following individuals for their assistance: Cara Hvisdas, Erika Gonzalez, and Ryan Brophy for their management and organization of the chapter content; Jordyn Bennett and April Billick for overseeing the layout; and John Bond for his guidance.

Last, but certainly not least, we would like to thank our families for allowing us to devote our time and energy toward completing this important and worthwhile project.

Terry Kim, MD
Derek W. DelMonte, MD
Preeya K. Gupta, MD

About the Editor

Terry Kim, MD, Professor of Ophthalmology at Duke University Eye Center in Durham, North Carolina, received his medical degree from Duke University School of Medicine in Durham and completed his residency and chief residency in ophthalmology at Emory Eye Center in Atlanta, Georgia. He continued with his fellowship training in corneal, external disease, and refractive surgery at Wills Eye Hospital in Philadelphia, Pennsylvania. He was then recruited to Duke University Eye Center, where he serves as principal and coinvestigator on a number of research grants from the National Institutes of Health and other institutions. Dr. Kim is a former director of the Residency Program and now serves as Director of Fellowship Programs.

Dr. Kim's academic accomplishments include his extensive publications in the peer-reviewed literature, which include more than 200 journal articles, textbook chapters, and scientific abstracts. He is also coauthor and coeditor of 2 well-respected textbooks on corneal diseases and cataract surgery. Dr. Kim has delivered more than 200 invited lectures, both nationally and internationally.

Dr. Kim was a recipient of the Achievement Award and the Senior Achievement Award from the American Academy of Ophthalmology (AAO). His clinical and research work earned him honors and grants from the National Institutes of Health, Fight for Sight/Research to Prevent Blindness, Heed Ophthalmic Foundation, Alcon Laboratories, and Allergan. Dr. Kim is listed continually in Best Doctors in America, Best Doctors in North Carolina, and America's Top Ophthalmologists. He has been voted by his peers as one of the 250 most prominent cataract and intraocular lens surgeons in the country by *Premier Surgeon*, as one of the "135 Leading Ophthalmologists in America" by Becker's ASC Review, as well as one of the "Top 50 Opinion Leaders" by *Cataract & Refractive Surgery Today*.

Dr. Kim serves on the Governing Board for the American Society of Cataract and Refractive Surgery (ASCRS) as Chair of the Cornea Clinical Committee, on the Annual Program Committee for the AAO, and on the Executive Committee and Board of Directors for the Cornea Society. He recently was inducted into the International Intra-Ocular Implant Club and is consultant to the Ophthalmic Devices Panel of the FDA. Kim also sits on the editorial board for several journals, including *Cornea, Journal of Cataract and Refractive Surgery, Ocular Surgery News, EyeWorld, Cataract & Refractive Surgery Today, Premier Surgeon, Review of Ophthalmology, Advanced Ocular Care,* and *Topics in Ocular Antiinfectives.* As consultant ophthalmologist for the Duke men's basketball team, Kim provides ophthalmic care for the players and coaches and has performed surgical procedures that have been featured on nationally televised programs such as those aired on the Discovery Channel.

About the Associate Editors

Derek W. DelMonte, MD received his medical degree from the University of Michigan in Ann Arbor and completed his residency in ophthalmology at the Duke University Eye Center in Durham, North Carolina. He completed his formal education with a fellowship in cornea, external disease, and refractive surgery at the Bascom Palmer Eye Institute in Miami, Florida. Dr. DelMonte currently serves as an assistant professor of ophthalmology for the Duke University Medical Center in Durham. He also maintains an appointment at the Durham Veterans Affairs Hospital, where he sees patients and participates in resident clinical and surgical education.

Dr. DelMonte has published numerous journal articles and book chapters on topics in corneal and cataract surgery. He was a winner of the *Ophthalmology Times* National Resident Writer's Award and received the Residents' Award for Fellow Teacher of the Year during his fellowship.

Preeya K. Gupta, MD received her undergraduate and medical degrees from Northwestern University in Evanston, Illinois and Chicago, Illinois, respectively. She completed her residency at the Duke University Eye Center in Durham, North Carolina and then completed a cornea and refractive surgery fellowship at Minnesota Eye Consultants in Minneapolis, Minnesota. Dr. Gupta is an assistant professor of ophthalmology at the Duke University Eye Center and currently is Clinical Medical Director of the Duke University Eye Center at Page Road.

Nationally, Dr. Gupta serves as an elected member of the ASCRS Young Physicians and Residents Clinical Committee. She is actively involved with clinical education and serves as faculty on the ASCRS Resident and Fellows Forum Committee. She also is an elected member of the Vanguard Ophthalmology Society.

Dr. Gupta has coauthored a number of book chapters and papers in the peer-reviewed literature. She serves as a reviewer for a number of journals, including the *American Journal of Ophthalmology* and *Journal of Refractive Surgery*.

Contributing Authors

Iqbal Ike K. Ahmed, MD, FRCSC (Question 32)
Assistant Professor of Ophthalmology
University of Toronto
Toronto, Ontario, Canada
Credit Valley Hospital
Mississauga, Ontario, Canada

Eric C. Amesbury, MD (Question 11)
Veterans Affairs
Palo Alto Health Care System
Palo Alto, California

Lisa Brothers Arbisser, MD (Question 22)
Cofounder
Eye Surgeons Associates, PC
Iowa and Illinois Quad Cities
Adjunct Associate Professor
John A. Moran Eye Center
University of Utah
Salt Lake City, Utah

Rosa Braga-Mele MD, MEd, FRCSC (Question 29)
Professor of Ophthalmology
University of Toronto
Director of Cataract Surgery
Kensington Eye Institute
Toronto, Ontario, Canada

David F. Chang, MD (Foreword, Question 20)
Clinical Professor of Ophthalmology
University of California, San Francisco
San Francisco, California

Steve Charles, MD, FACS, FICS (Question 5)
Clinical Professor of Ophthalmology
University of Tennessee
Charles Retina Institute
Memphis, Tennessee

Theodore J. Christakis, MD (Question 29)
University of Toronto
Toronto, Ontario, Canada

Fred Chu, MD (Question 13)
Rush University Medical Center
Chicago, Illinois

Robert J. Cionni, MD (Question 38)
Cincinnati Eye Institute
Cincinnati, Ohio

Garry P. Condon, MD (Question 48)
Associate Professor of Ophthalmology
Drexel University College of Medicine
Philadelphia, Pennsylvania
Chairman
Department of Ophthalmology
Allegheny General Hospital
Clinical Assistant Professor of
  Ophthalmology
University of Pittsburgh
Pittsburgh, Pennsylvania

Alan S. Crandall, MD (Question 49)
Professor and Senior Vice Chair
Director of Glaucoma and Cataract
Co-Director
Moran International Division
John A. Moran Eye Center
University of Utah
Salt Lake City, Utah

Mahshad Darvish, MD (Question 10)
Cincinnati Eye Institute
Cincinnati, Ohio

Uday Devgan, MD (Question 39)
Devgan Eye Surgery
Los Angeles and Beverly Hills, California
Chief of Ophthalmology
Olive View UCLA Medical Center
Associate Clinical Professor
Jules Stein Eye Institute
University of California School of
  Medicine
Los Angeles, California

Dipanjal Dey, MD (Question 16)
Consultant
Cataract, Cornea and External Eye
    Diseases
Medical Director
Alipurduar Lions Eye Bank
Alipurduar Lions Eye Hospital
Alipurduar, West Bengal, India

Deepinder K. Dhaliwal, MD, LAc (Question 2)
Associate Professor of Ophthalmology
UPMC Eye Center
The Eye and Ear Institute
University of Pittsburgh School of
    Medicine
Pittsburgh, PA

Paul Ernest, MD (Question 18)
Cataract and Refractive Specialist
TLC Eyecare & Laser Centers of Michigan
Jackson, Michigan

William J. Fishkind, MD, FACS (Question 25)
Clinical Professor
University of Utah
Salt Lake City, Utah
Clinical Professor
University of Arizona
Fishkind & Bakewell Eye Care and Surgery
    Center
Tucson, Arizona

Nicole R. Fram, MD (Question 46)
Advanced Vision Care
Los Angeles, California

Scott Greenbaum, MD (Question 19)
Assistant Clinical Professor
Department of Ophthalmology
New York University
Attending Surgeon
Manhattan Eye, Ear and Throat Hospital
New York, New York

David R. Hardten, MD (Question 7)
Director of Refractive Surgery
Minnesota Eye Consultants, PA
Minneapolis, Minnesota

Mojgan Hassanlou, MD FRCSC (Question 2)
Director of Cornea and External Disease
Cornea, Refractive, Cataract Surgery
Herzig Eye Institute
Toronto, Ontario, Canada

Bonnie An Henderson, MD (Question 15)
Ophthalmic Consultants of Boston
Clinical Professor of Ophthalmology
Tufts University School of Medicine
Boston, Massachusetts

Warren E. Hill, MD, FACS (Question 9)
Medical Director
East Valley Ophthalmology
Mesa, Arizona

Richard S. Hoffman, MD (Question 34)
Clinical Associate Professor of
    Ophthalmology
Oregon Health and Science University
Eugene, Oregon

Edward Holland, MD (Question 10)
Cincinnati Eye Institute
Cincinnati, Ohio

Sumitra Khandelwal, MD (Question 7)
Assistant Professor of Ophthalmology
Baylor College of Medicine
Houston, Texas

Gaston O. Lacayo III, MD (Question 47)
Assistant Professor of Ophthalmology
Rush University Medical Center
Chicago, Illinos
Assistant Clinical Professor of
    Ophthalmology
Florida International University
Miami, Florida

Stephen S. Lane, MD (Question 45)
Adjunct Professor of Ophthalmology
University of Minnesota
Minneapolis, Minnesota
Medical Director
Associated Eye Care
Stillwater, Minnesota

Richard A. Lewis, MD (Question 41)
Consultant
Sacramento Surgical Eye Consultants
Sacramento, California

Richard L. Lindstrom, MD (Question 7)
Founder and Attending Surgeon
Minnesota Eye Consultants
Adjunct Professor Emeritus
University of Minnesota
Minneapolis, Minnesota

Brian Little, MA, DO, FHEA, FRCS, FRCOphth (Question 23)
Consultant Ophthalmologist
Training Director, Cataract Service
National Health Service
Moorfields Eye Hospital NHS Foundation Trust
Private Practice
London Medical
London, England

Francis S. Mah, MD (Question 40)
Director
Cornea and External Disease
Co-Director
Refractive Surgery
Scripps Clinic
La Jolla, California

Parag Majmudar, MD (Question 13)
Associate Professor of Ophthalmology
Rush University Medical Center
Chicago, Illinois

Boris Malyugin, MD, PhD (Question 21)
Professor of Ophthalmology
Department of Cataract and Implant Surgery
Deputy Director General (R&D, Edu)
S. Fyodorov Eye Microsurgery Complex
Moscow, Russia

Nick Mamalis, MD (Question 42)
Professor of Ophthalmology
Co-Director
Intermountain Ocular Research Center
Director
Ocular Pathology
John A. Moran Eye Center
University of Utah Medical Center
Salt Lake City, Utah

Samuel Masket, MD (Question 46)
Advanced Vision Care
Los Angeles, California

Kevin M. Miller, MD (Question 11)
Kolokotrones Professor of Clinical Ophthalmology
Jules Stein Eye Institute
Los Angeles, California

Christina S. Moon, MD (Question 30)
Clinical Instructor
Bascom Palmer Eye Institute
Miller School of Medicine
University of Miami
Miami, Florida

Kristiana D. Neff, MD (Question 3)
Carolina Cataract & Laser Center
Charleston, South Carolina

Louis D. "Skip" Nichamin, MD (Question 33)
Medical Director
Laurel Eye Clinic, LLP
Brookville, Pennsylvania

Thomas A. Oetting, MS, MD (Question 31)
Professor of Clinical Ophthalmology and
    Director
Ophthalmology Residency Program
University of Iowa
Chief of Eye Service
Deputy Director of Surgery Service
Veterans Affairs Medical Center
Iowa City, Iowa

Randall J. Olson, MD (Question 26)
Professor and Chair
Department of Ophthalmology and Visual
    Sciences
University of Utah
CEO
John A. Moran Eye Center
Salt Lake City, Utah

Robert H. Osher, MD (Question 36)
Professor of Ophthalmology
University of Cincinnati
Medical Director Emeritus
Cincinnati Eye Institute
Cincinnati, Ohio

Mark Packer, MD, FACS, CPI (Question 24)
Associate Clinical Professor
Oregon Health & Science University
Portland, Oregon
Bowie Vision Institute, LLC for
    Ophthalmic Research
Bowie, Maryland

Mauricio A. Perez, MD (Question 14)
Cincinnati Eye Institute
University of Cincinnati
Cincinnati, Ohio

Michael B. Raizman, MD (Question 43)
Ophthalmic Consultants of Boston
Associate Professor of Ophthalmology
Tufts University School of Medicine
Boston, Massachusetts

Thomas Samuelson, MD (Question 4)
Attending Surgeon
Minnesota Eye Consultants and Phillips
    Eye Institute
Adjunct Associate Professor
University of Minnesota
Minneapolis, Minnesota

Barry Seibel, MD (Question 28)
Clinical Assistant Professor of
    Ophthalmology
UCLA Geffen School of Medicine
Seibel Vision Surgery
Los Angeles, California

Eric J. Sigler, MD (Question 5)
Charles Retina Institute
Memphis, Tennessee

Michael E. Snyder, MD (Question 14)
Board of Directors
Cincinnati Eye Institute
Volunteer Assistant Professor
University of Cincinnati
Cincinnati, Ohio

Roger F. Steinert, MD (Question 27)
Irving H. Leopold Professor of
    Ophthalmology
Chair of the Department of
    Ophthalmology
Director of the Gavin Herbert Eye Institute
Professor of Biomedical Engineering
University of California, Irvine
Irvine, California

Geoffrey C. Tabin, MA, MD (Question 16)
Professor of Ophthalmology and Visual
    Sciences
John A. Moran Eye Center
University of Utah Medical School
Salt Lake City, Utah
Chairman
Himalayan Cataract Project
Waterbury, Vermont

Benjamin Thomas, MD (Question 16)
International Ophthalmology Fellow
John A. Moran Eye Center
University of Utah Medical School
Salt Lake City, Utah

Richard Tipperman, MD (Question 17)
Attending Surgeon
Wills Eye Hospital
Philadelphia, Pennsylvania

William Trattler, MD (Question 47)
Center for Excellence in Eye Care
Miami, Florida

Farrell C. Tyson, MD, FACS (Question 6)
Medical Director, CEO
Cape Coral Eye Center/Tyson Eye
Cape Coral and Fort Myers, Florida

Robin R. Vann, MD (Question 8)
Assistant Professor of Ophthalmology
Duke University School of Medicine
Chief
Comprehensive Service
Duke Eye Center
Durham, North Carolina

David T. Vroman, MD (Question 3)
Founding Partner
Carolina Cataract & Laser Center
Medical Director
Lifepoint Ocular Division
Charleston and Ladson, South Carolina

R. Bruce Wallace III, MD (Question 12)
Clinical Director of Ophthalmology
Tulane Medical School
Clinical Director of Ophthalmology
LSU School of Medicine
New Orleans, Louisiana
Medical Director
Wallace Eye Surgery & Wallace Laser &
    Surgery Center
Alexandria, Louisiana

Keith A. Warren, MD (Question 44)
President and CEO
Warren Retina Associates
Overland Park, Kansas
Clinical Professor of Ophthalmology
University of Kansas
Lawrence, Kansas

Sonia H. Yoo, MD (Question 30)
Professor of Ophthalmology
Bascom Palmer Eye Institute
University of Miami
Miller School of Medicine
Miami, Florida

Preface

In today's age of information, we must deal with an overwhelming overload of material from emails, text messages, and the internet in general, as well as more traditional sources of television, radio, and print media. As busy clinicians, we have the daunting task of sorting through peer-reviewed journal articles, textbook chapters, trade journals, and content from international, national, regional, and local meetings and webinars in an attempt to extract the important, up-to-date, and clinically relevant information we feel will benefit our patients and practices.

However, one of the most valuable and trusted sources of information still comes from talking to your peers and colleagues. In medicine, the term for this exchange of information was coined *curbside consult* and is a commonplace occurrence in every specialty of medicine, including ophthalmology. This is when a busy practitioner, faced with a diagnostic or treatment question or dilemma, solicits practical advice from a trusted and knowledgeable expert in the field. These brief consultations take place every day in clinic hallways, over the telephone, at meetings, and by email. The query is brief and concise. The response is practical, to the point, and based on that expert's knowledge, judgement, and experience.

This textbook on cataract surgery seeks to provide a compendium of this information—answers to 49 of the most clinically relevant and commonly posed questions to specialists by practicing colleagues. This educational question-and-answer format remains unique among other publications. Just as a curbside consult is distinguished from a lecture or an instructional course, so is this compilation different from a scientific journal or standard textbook. Most of these clinical questions do not individually merit a lecture, review article, or book chapter, and are not answered definitively by the scientific literature.

With this second edition, my associate editors and I worked hard to revise, update, and improve the content from the first edition of *Curbside Consultation in Cataract Surgery*, which was conceived and edited by Dr. David F. Chang. We knew we had a formidable challenge ahead of us, due to the high standard and level of perfection that David achieves with every task he undertakes. As a result, we injected fresh content into this second edition with respect to new topics and questions, up-to-date responses, and more diagrams, figures, and tables that are both instructive and easy to reference. We invited different cataract consultants to answer the popular questions carried over from the first edition to get some fresh perspective. We also invited new faculty to join our esteemed list of 49 cataract experts from the United States and abroad.

In an effort to facilitate the search for topics, we divided the book into 3 sections: preoperative, intraoperative, and postoperative questions. The advice from our surgical consultants is based upon their personal experience, their review of the evidence-based literature, and, in some cases, their own clinical studies. As with the 1st edition, we asked that our consultants' answers meet David's original proposed criteria of content: the 4 "Cs." The advice must be current (timely), concise (summarizing), credible (evidence-based), and clinically relevant (practical).

In addition to the paperback format, we are excited to offer this textbook in digital format as well. Whether you are thumbing through the pages of the paperback or swiping through the pages of the digital book on your tablet, we feel confident you will find the content to be easily accessible and manageable. Regardless of whether you read the first edition or are reading this new edition for the first time, we hope you appreciate the spirit and value of this unique "curbside consult" educational format and feel that you truly have the expert advice of our specialists right at your fingertips. With the hectic schedules and time constraints we face as clinicians, we feel this reference will be a very practical and time-efficient resource for the questions you face in your cataract practice. On behalf of my associate editors and contributing authors, we sincerely hope you enjoy this textbook and find it helpful in improving the care of your patients.

Terry Kim, MD

Foreword

When it was published in 2007, the first edition of *Curbside Consultation in Cataract Surgery: 49 Clinical Questions* launched a new series of ophthalmic subspecialty textbooks compiled in a reader-friendly, question-and-answer format. The popular *Curbside Consultation* series now includes editions for glaucoma, neuro-ophthalmology, retina, oculoplastics, uveitis, and corneal and external disease, with a refractive-surgery version in development.

This *Curbside Consultation* is the first title in the series to be updated with a second edition, and I am delighted that my original and very capable associate editor, Terry Kim, has assumed the mantle of editor. Terry is a gifted teacher and is one of the most respected cornea, refractive, and cataract surgeons in the world. He is joined by two of his colleagues and rising anterior-segment stars from Duke, Preeya Gupta and Derek DelMonte. Together, this impressive team has done a wonderful job of revising and updating this practical textbook.

Readers of the second edition will find that more than half of the clinical questions and the consultants are new, whereas the retained chapters have been fully updated, often with new authors. I am very impressed with the new questions posed by the editors, as well as with the many new experts they recruited as consultants. The result is a fresh approach that successfully zeros in on the most vexing and relevant clinical issues that cataract surgeons currently face.

The current edition still retains the features that have made SLACK's *Curbside Consultation* series so popular: practical questions that are not always addressed in print or from the podium, succinct explanations that highlight the bottom line, consultations from experts who know both the literature and the art, and a convenient way for ophthalmologists to quickly look up concise information on the spot.

This new edition succeeds in surpassing the quality of the original and will appeal to all cataract surgeons, from residents-in-training to experienced, higher volume surgeons. Whether read cover-to-cover or used as a desktop reference when a specific question arises, the second edition of *Curbside Consultation in Cataract Surgery* is a valuable resource that every cataract surgeon will appreciate.

David F. Chang, MD
Clinical Professor of Ophthalmology
University of California, San Francisco
San Francisco, California
Altos Eye Physicians
Los Altos, California

SECTION I

PREOPERATIVE QUESTIONS

My Patient Has Dry Eye and Blepharitis. How and When Do I Need to Treat These Conditions Before Cataract Surgery?

Preeya K. Gupta, MD

Dry eye affects millions of Americans and is one of the most frequent reasons for seeking eye care. The prevalence of dry eye has been studied in a variety of populations and is more common in older adults and women.[1,2] The prevalence of dry eye has been reported to be greater than 10% of the population.[3]

Similar to dry eye, blepharitis and meibomian gland dysfunction are also highly prevalent and underrecognized. A large interview-based study by Lemp and Nichols[4] found that 32% of their study-population patients reported at least 1 symptom of blepharitis or dry eye and experienced this at least 50% of the time in the prior 12 months. Clearly, there is significant disease burden in our general population. Early recognition and treatment are the keys to success.

Dry eye can be classified into 2 major categories: aqueous-deficient and evaporative dry eye.[5] Identifying which type of dry eye your patient suffers from is necessary to choose the correct treatment.

Aqueous-deficient dry eye is secondary to poor production of tears from the lacrimal gland. In my clinical experience, I find this to be less common than evaporative dry eye syndrome. Often, patients with aqueous deficiency have a coincident autoimmune or systemic inflammatory condition.

Evaporative dry eye syndrome is secondary to poor secretion and altered composition of meibum from the meibomian glands. The thick secretions do not flow readily into the tear film, resulting in excessive evaporation and hyperosmolarity of the tears, thus increasing ocular surface inflammation.

Given the above, odds are that a patient above the age of 65 years who is coming to see you for cataract surgery has some degree of dry eye or blepharitis. However, both dry eye and blepharitis are often overlooked and undertreated by physicans.[6] I believe that, in the era of refractive cataract surgery, where patients have high expectations with respect to refractive outcomes, it is vital to identify and address these conditions prior to pursuing cataract surgery.

Clinical History

SYMPTOMS

Patients with dry eye and blepharitis may complain of red and irritated eyes, crusting on the eyelids and lashes, frequent stye formation, or having an overall reddish hue to the eyelid margins. Uncontrolled blepharitis alters the lipid composition of the meibomian gland secretions, making the oil more viscous and thus poorly secreted. These oils are essential to maintaining tear viscosity and stability. Alteration in this pathway negatively affects tear-film barrier function and causes excessive evaporation of tears, therefore impairing overall vision quality.

Asking your patient the following few simple screening questions can help you to determine the severity of dry eye:

1. How often do you notice that your eyes are red, irritated, and tired?

2. Are your symptoms worse at the end of the day or with prolonged reading?

3. How often do you use artificial tears?

By asking these questions, you can confirm that the patient suffers from common symptoms, such as redness or irritation, and get a sense of how severe the problem is by determining how often they choose to pursue treatment for it.

Clinical Examination

Performing a detailed slit-lamp examination can allow the surgeon to easily identify a patient who may be vulnerable to, or suffer from, dry eye. Patients may be asymptomatic preoperatively, but dry eye can be exacerbated by surgery in an individual who is at risk.

KEY COMPONENTS

1. Slit-lamp examination:

   a. *External:* Look for signs of comorbid conditions, eg, rosacea, seborrheic dermatitis, or signs of autoimmune diseases such as lupus (malar rash), thyroid dysfunction (brittle nails, dry skin, hair loss), or Sjögren's syndrome (dry mouth, enlarged parotid glands).

   b. *Eyelid position:* Look for any signs of ectropion or lagophthalmos, which could allow for excessive tear evaporation.

   c. *Meibomian glands and lid margin:* Apply gentle pressure to the lid margin to observe oil flow from the meibomian glands. Dysfunctional glands will have thick or toothpaste-like secretions. Assess for lid margin vascularity and posterior dragging of the gland orifice (Figure 1-1).

   d. *Tear film:* A tear film height <1 mm, tear break-up time <10 seconds, or foamy tears can signify poor tear film quality.

   e. *Cornea:* Fluorescein staining can easily reveal punctate erosions, and observing the pattern of staining can be helpful (ie, inferior staining should signal the observer to search for causes of lagophthalmos or exposure, whereas a diffuse pattern of staining is more common with poor tear production and excessive tear evaporation due to meibomian gland dysfunction).

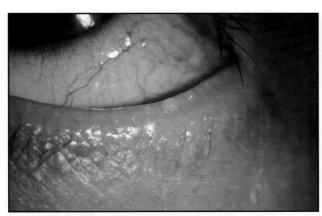

Figure 1-1. Thick secretions elicited with gentle pressure applied along the lid margin and meibomian glands. Note extensive lid margin vascularity, which is consistent with ocular rosacea.

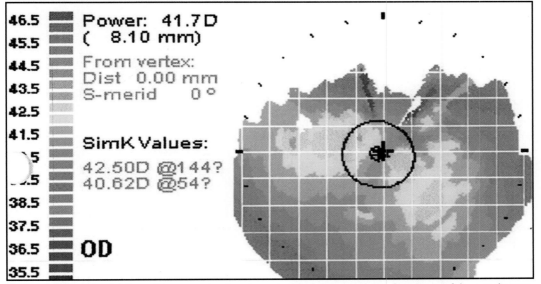

Figure 1-2. Placido disk-based topography showing missing data superiorly, suggestive of dry eye disease.

2. Topography: Imaging of the cornea with a Placido disk-based topographer can be a good screening tool. Often, patients with dry eye and blepharitis will have missing data (Figure 1-2).

3. Schirmer testing: Although not necessarily the most reliable test, it can be used as a screening tool to determine whether basal tear production is below average (ie, <10 mm in 5 minutes).

Treatment

Treatment of dry eye and meibomian gland dysfunction are very important, especially prior to cataract surgery. In my practice, I treat patients with evaporative dry eye differently than those with aqueous-deficient dry eye.

For nearly all of my patients with dry eye, regardless of the type, I recommend using preservative-free artificial tears every 2 to 4 hours, as tolerated; a lubricating gel or ointment at bedtime;

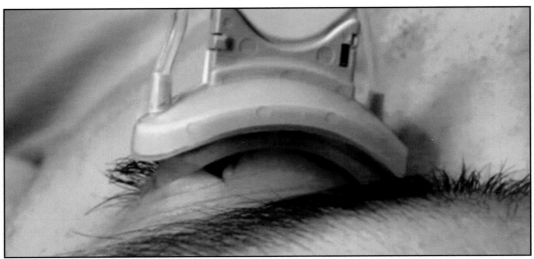

Figure 1-3. LipiFlow thermal pulsation device placed between eyelids in treating a patient with significant meibomian gland dysfunction.

and warm compresses to the eyelids 2 to 3 times per day. For those patients with largely aqueous-deficient dry eye, we also discuss starting cyclosporine, 0.05% (RESTASIS) twice daily. If the condition is severe, a short course of topical steroids may also be considered.

For those patients with primarily evaporative dry eye and meibomian gland dysfunction, in addition to the previous instructions, I ask patients to scrub eyelids with baby shampoo or pre-medicated cleansing pads. We also discuss the option of starting topical azithromycin (AzaSite) applied directly to the eye lids once daily to improve blepharitis symptoms or starting oral doxy-cycline (50 to 100 mg daily). Some patients also have reported improved dry eye symptoms with use of omega-3 fatty acid supplements, taken twice daily in doses of 1500 mg.

For those individuals with moderate to severe evaporative dry eye, I also discuss the option of LipiFlow (TearScience) or Intense Pulsed Light (DermaMed Solutions, LLC) therapy (Figures 1-3 and 1-4). Both treatments are aimed at improving the health of the meibomian glands, allowing the formation of a better meibum and allowing the lipid to reach the tear film, to increase tear stability. Both treatments are tolerated well and have achieved good results in my practice.

Regardless of the treatment methods chosen, it is crucial to achieve good control of any ocular surface disease prior to proceeding with surgery. The time taken to treat these conditions preoperatively will help any surgeon to achieve more accurate intraocular lens calculations and decrease the risk of postoperative infections. It also will allow the patient to have realistic expectations and ensure a better outcome after surgery.

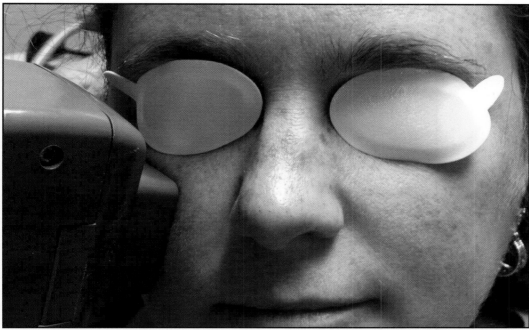

Figure 1-4. Intense pulsed-light therapy in the treatment of evaporative dry eye disease. The hand piece plate is placed onto the skin surface after the eyes are covered appropriately with protective shields. The light is applied from one tragus to the other, encompassing the lower eyelids and cheeks.

References

1. Lemp MA. Epidemiology and classification of dry eye. *Adv Exp Med Biol.* 1998;438:791-803.
2. Schaumberg DA, Sullivan DA, Buring JE, Dana MR. Prevalence of dry eye syndrome among US women. *Am J Ophthalmol.* 2003;136(2):318-326.
3. Moss SE, Klein R, Klein BE. Prevalence of and risk factors for dry eye syndrome. *Arch Ophthalmol.* 2000;118(9):1264-1268.
4. Lemp MA, Nichols KK. Blepharitis in the United States 2009: a survey-based perspective on prevalence and treatment. *Ocul Surf.* 2009;7(2):S1-S14.
5. The definition and classification of dry eye disease: report of the Definition and Classification Subcommittee of the International Dry Eye WorkShop (2007). *Ocul Surf.* 2007;5(2):75-92.
6. Lin IC, Gupta PK, Boehlke CS, Lee PP. Documentation of conformance to preferred practice patterns in caring for patients with dry eye. *Arch Ophthalmol.* 2010;128(5):619-623.

My Patient Has Unreliable Topography Due to Ocular Surface Pathology. What Are My Options for Treatment and Intraocular Lens Selection?

Deepinder K. Dhaliwal, MD, LAc and
Mojgan Hassanlou, MD, FRCSC

The most common cause of unreliable topography due to corneal surface irregularity in our cataract population is epithelial basement membrane dystrophy. Salzmann's nodular degeneration and subepithelial scarring are seen less commonly. The resulting irregular corneal astigmatism can result in poor best-corrected distance visual acuity postcataract surgery and difficulty with proper intraocular lens (IOL) selection. It is critical to identify such patients properly and to treat them appropriately to achieve optimal results from cataract procedures. It is especially important in patients who are considering a premium IOL, as their expectation for crisp, uncorrected vision postoperatively is high.

Identification

The first step is identification. Although it is easier to visualize Salzmann's nodules on the cornea, epithelial basement membrane dystrophy can be missed with the slit beam. A simple and quick diagnostic test is to place fluorescein in the eye and examine the cornea with broad illumination under blue light. Subtle corneal irregularity can be seen as areas of negative staining (Figure 2-1). It is important not to use Fluress (Akorn Inc) (fluorescein sodium and benoxinate hydrochloride ophthalmic solution) or other such combination anesthetic or fluorescein drops, as these thicker drops can mask subtle, underlying corneal pathology. We simply moisten a fluorescein strip with proparacaine or balanced salt solution and place the strip just inside the lower lid on the tarsal conjunctiva. After the patient blinks a few times, areas of negative staining can be seen quite easily with diffuse blue illumination.

Figure 2-1. Corneal irregularity can be seen as areas of negative staining with fluorescein application.

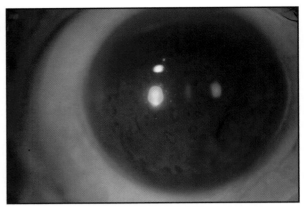

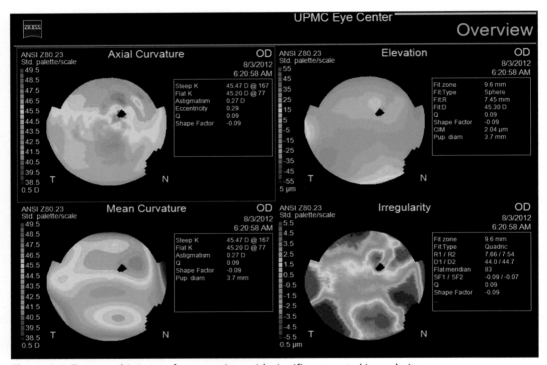

Figure 2-2. Topographic image from a patient with significant central irregularity.

Treatment

If the areas of irregularity are within the visual axis, we assess the visual impact by performing corneal topography and keratometry. If the mires are significantly irregular or if there is central irregularity on the topography (Figure 2-2), we recommend a corneal resurfacing procedure prior to cataract surgery.

We also ask the patient about symptoms of recurrent erosion on awakening. If there have been episodes of corneal erosion, we treat it with a hypertonic saline ointment, such as Muro 128 5% ointment (sodium chloride hypertonicity ophthalmic ointment, 5%), nightly. If there is no improvement after 4 to 6 weeks of conservative treatment, we then proceed with corneal resurfacing.

Corneal resurfacing is performed by removing the irregular epithelium with a spatula or blade, but care has to be taken not to damage the underlying corneal tissue. We then prefer to do a light excimer laser application (phototherapeutic keratectomy), removing only 1 to 3 microns of tissue, or use a diamond burr.[1,2] These modalities improve epithelial adhesion; therefore, they are important in patients with irregular astigmatism and recurrent erosion. In cases of central irregular astigmatism alone, the central corneal epithelium can be removed without additional treatment. Pathology such as Salzmann's nodules is treated by first removing the overlying epithelium and then debulking manually as much of the nodule as possible. In almost all cases, an edge can be lifted with a spatula; then the nodule can be peeled off the cornea with forceps.

In all cases, a bandage contact lens is placed in the eye and patients are asked to use topical steroids, such as fluoromethalone 0.1% 4 times daily and broad-spectrum topical antibiotics 4 times daily. Topical nonsteroidal anti-inflammatory drugs may also be used for pain control over the first 24 to 48 hours, at appropriate labeled dosing. Preservative-free artificial tears are used 4 times daily as well, staggered 2 hours after the medicated drops; therefore, the patient is placing drops in the eye every 2 hours, which greatly aids in keeping the ocular surface moist to optimize healing. Epithelial healing is monitored through the bandage contact lens, which is kept in place as long as a defect remains, typically for 3 to 5 days.

If there is a delay in epithelial healing, consideration should be given to punctal plug placement and use of oral doxycycline or azithromycin. The topical steroid is tapered by one drop each week, and the antibiotic is discontinued after complete re-epithelialization. After bandage contact lens removal, the patient is advised to use hypertonic saline ointment nightly, to aid in stability of the newly regenerated corneal epithelium.

The ocular surface is generally stable in 6 to 8 weeks, at which time topography and keratometry are repeated. At this time, we can assess the patient's interest and suitability for a toric IOL, which is indicated for regular corneal astigmatism, not for irregular astigmatism, or a multifocal or accommodating IOL. We have found this approach helpful, as surface corneal irregularity is identified and treated before cataract surgery, and any hyperopic shift after phototherapeutic keratectomy can be offset by proper IOL selection.

References

1. Aldave AJ, Kamal KM, Vo RC, Yu F. Epithelial debridement and Bowman's layer polishing for visually significant epithelial irregularity and recurrent corneal erosions. *Cornea.* 2009;28(10):1085-1090.
2. Sridhar MS, Rapuano CJ, Cosar CB, Cohen EJ, Laibson PR. Phototherapeutic keratectomy versus diamond burr polishing of Bowman's membrane in the treatment of recurrent corneal erosions associated with anterior basement membrane dystrophy. *Ophthalmology.* 2002;109(4):674-679.

QUESTION

WHEN AND HOW SHOULD CATARACT SURGERY ALONE BE PERFORMED IN PATIENTS WITH FUCHS' DYSTROPHY?

David T. Vroman, MD and
Kristiana D. Neff, MD

Making decisions regarding cataract surgery in the Fuchs' dystrophy patient has become more challenging in the era of Descemet's stripping endothelial keratoplasty (EK), Descemet's membrane endothelial keratoplasty (DMEK), and evolving cataract technology. In years past, cataract surgery prior to performing penetrating keratoplasty (PK) often could achieve acceptable vision, in the range of 20/40 to 20/50, and postpone the need for a full-thickness transplant. In addition, the surgical complexity of a full-thickness transplant, the healing rate, and the final visual potential were not affected by the timing of cataract surgery. In eyes with frank corneal decompensation, PK and cataract were performed together.

Endothelial keratoplasty significantly changed this paradigm. Visual acuity outcomes after EK and EK/cataract are usually better than 20/40, and 20/20 outcomes are common. In addition, earlier corneal surgery probably results in better long-term visual acuity, especially if anterior stromal haze is developing, which will remain after EK.

In the PK era, cataract and corneal surgeons might lean toward cataract surgery prior to PK in borderline cases, whereas in the EK era, earlier corneal surgery is more common. Despite the excellent results in EK and EK/cataract combined surgery, there are still patients where determining the correct surgical course is challenging.

Variables to Consider

Many variables are considered when deciding to perform cataract surgery in a Fuchs' dystrophy patient. The patient's history and his or her visual demands must be weighed primarily. Is the patient a 90-year-old with limited activities who will function well with central guttae, trace edema, and vision of 20/50? Or is the patient a demanding surgeon who pilots planes as a hobby and needs to achieve maximal clarity as soon as possible, with the fewest days away from work?

Obviously, most patients fall somewhere in between and weighing these intangible variables is difficult.

Postoperative care of the eye is also an important variable, as patients undergoing EK require prolonged steroid use and the ability to seek medical care for signs of an implant rejection. A historical clue that may suggest benefit in performing a combined surgery is whether the patient experiences morning blur that clears through the day. This reveals that the patient's endothelium is compromised enough that simply having the eyes closed overnight overwhelms the pump function, leading to morning epithelial cell edema (ie, microcystic edema).

Determining the Surgical Plan

The examination is the next most important component in determining the surgical plan. Several important findings will increase consideration for combined cataract and corneal surgery.

Obvious stromal or epithelial edema, even outside of the visual axis, will require corneal transplantation to resolve. Anterior stromal haze below Bowman's layer suggests collagen changes that will persist after cataract surgery alone and that can progress without EK. This finding can occur earlier than might be expected, and earlier EK may prevent progression and sometimes diminish this haze.

The severity of the guttae and the status of Descemet's membrane are important. Even in patients without edema, confluent guttae can cause glare and decrease contrast sensitivity. Unfortunately, it is sometimes impossible to know whether glare is due primarily to the cataract or the guttae. Descemet's membrane itself can sometimes become opaque. This is uncommon, but it can occur prior to significant accumulation of stromal edema. These membranes can be thick and tough when removed at surgery.

Finally, the density of the cataract may play a role in the decision. A very dense cataract will be more difficult to remove and likely will cause more endothelial damage than one that is of moderate density.

Ancillary testing can be beneficial in some situations. Pachymetry is especially useful if there is documented corneal thickening over time or if there is significant asymmetry between eyes. These eyes likely will benefit from a combined surgery. Unfortunately, no specific pachymetric cutoff can determine which path to take because there is a wide range of normal. A cornea with normal pachymetry of 475 μm is significantly edematous at 550 μm, whereas another cornea could normally measure 600 μm and be edema free.

Specular microscopy can also be beneficial in some situations. For patients with confluent guttae, or early edema, cell counts probably do not play a role in the surgical decision making. Typically, these images reveal few or no cells centrally. For patients followed over time, cell counts can be beneficial in seeing trends and educating the patient.

After the patient's visual demands, history, slit-lamp examination, and ancillary testing are evaluated, a decision on surgical intervention is made. If cataract surgery alone is deemed most appropriate, the surgeon can take steps to ensure an optimal outcome. The goal is to protect the remaining endothelium maximally during surgery.

The use of viscoelastics is critical. A dispersive viscoelastic with a low viscosity will spread through the anterior chamber and provide a protective coating for the endothelium. Use of a cohesive under the dispersive agent, ie, the soft-shell technique, forces the dispersive viscoelastic to the endothelium. The soft-shell technique has been shown to be protective, and it preserves endothelial cells.[1]

The surgical technique should minimize phacoemulsification time and power. A manual approach to nuclear disassembly, such as prechop or phaco chop, can minimize ultrasound damage. Use of advanced modalities, such as torsional or transversal ultrasound, can increase the efficiency of lens removal and decrease total energy dissipated in the eye. Emergence of femtosecond lasers, to assist in lens fragmentation, has reduced the total ultrasound energy required for cataract removal, and this may prove beneficial to Fuchs' dystrophy patients as well.[2]

Several other considerations warrant preoperative planning. If there is a significant concern for endothelial failure, yet cataract surgery alone is attempted, consideration of a myopic goal of −0.75 to −1.25 diopters could offset the typical hyperopic shift of a future Descemet's stripping EK. The goals and visual demands of the patient must be considered, as this will result in loss of uncorrected distance acuity, and this may not be an acceptable outcome for some patients. Furthermore, DMEK does not appear to create the same level of hyperopic shift. Knowing what corneal treatments are available in your region, if you are referring to a corneal surgeon following cataract surgery, could affect the desired refractive target.

Lens choice is another consideration. Use of toric intraocular lenses (IOLs) appears to be safe, although topography can be inaccurate if there is any stromal edema. Use of multifocal IOLs should be approached cautiously, as even minimal stromal edema or guttae can degrade the optical quality of the cornea. Frank stromal edema, after a multifocal implant, may be best treated with DMEK to minimize hyperopic shift and increase the chance of achieving 20/20 corneal clarity.

Postoperative Care

Finally, postoperative care may be tailored to the Fuchs' dystrophy patient. Use of a potent topical corticosteroid, such as difluprednate 0.05%, may be beneficial to the endothelium. Use of sodium chloride 5% may help clear small amounts of edema early postoperatively. If postcataract surgery edema persists past 6 weeks, preparation for EK is appropriate. Waiting many months with corneal edema can lead to permanent damage of the anterior cornea and limit final visual outcomes; therefore, early referral to a corneal specialist is more important than ever before.

Conclusion

Patients with Fuchs' dystrophy and cataract should be approached more thoughtfully than a patient with only cataracts. The patient's history, postoperative demands, ocular examination, and ancillary testing will suggest a prudent surgical course. When cataract surgery alone is undertaken, special surgical maneuvers and techniques can maximize the potential for a good outcome. Intraocular lens selection and target postoperative refraction may be affected by the level of Fuchs' dystrophy disease. When the endothelium fails, despite all precaution, early referral for EK is essential.

References

1. Tarnawska D, Wylegala E. Effectiveness of the soft-shell technique in patients with Fuchs' endothelial dystrophy. *J Cataract Refract Surg.* 2007;33:1907-1912.
2. Takács AI, Kovács I, Miháltz K, et al. Central corneal volume and endothelial cell count following femtosecond laser-assisted refractive cataract surgery compared to conventional phacoemulsification. *J Refract Surg.* 2012;28(6):387-391.

MY PATIENT HAS A CATARACT AND GLAUCOMA. WHICH PATIENTS NEED A COMBINED GLAUCOMA PROCEDURE, AND WHICH DEVICE(S) SHOULD I USE?

Thomas Samuelson, MD

The native crystalline lens, an important element of narrow- and closed-angle glaucoma, is becoming an increasingly important consideration in the management of adult-onset, open-angle glaucoma. There is compelling evidence that removal of a cataract improves intraocular pressure (IOP) control in patients with elevated IOP.[1-3] Moreover, recently approved microinvasive glaucoma procedures have been conceived specifically to combine with clear corneal phacoemulsification to augment the IOP-lowering effect of cataract extraction safely and synergistically and to reduce the number of medications necessary to control IOP. Accordingly, perhaps one of the first questions clinicians must address when managing a patient with glaucoma and uncontrolled IOP is, "What is the status of the crystalline lens?"

Clinical Challenges

The presentation of coincident cataract and glaucoma is one of the most common clinical challenges facing the anterior segment surgeon. Although the only effective therapeutic intervention for a cataract is surgical, glaucoma may be managed effectively either medically or surgically. As such, when you make the decision to intervene surgically for a cataract in a patient with established glaucoma, you also must determine whether to continue medical management of the glaucoma or perform combined cataract and glaucoma surgery.

Recent advances in the medical management of glaucoma have significantly reduced the number of traditional combined glaucoma procedures—phacoemulsification and trabeculectomy—that are performed. Better glaucoma medications have led to an increase in the percentage of patients who may be managed with cataract surgery alone. Further, it is now generally accepted that cataract surgery alone lowers IOP at least transiently in many, if not most, cases.

Perhaps the most compelling evidence of this fact is data from 2 important clinical trials, the Ocular Hypertension Treatment Study and the US Food and Drug Administration trial involving the iStent Trabecular Micro-Bypass stent (Glaukos Corporation).[1,2] Both of these trials demonstrate that cataract extraction alone lowers IOP. As such, cataract extraction alone is a viable option for many patients with both cataract and glaucoma. Even so, evidence suggests that combining cataract extraction with a microstent placed within Schlemm's canal significantly reduces the amount of medication needed postoperatively. Further, in the FDA premarket approval investigational device exemption trial, the safety profile of the iStent implanted at the time of cataract surgery was not significantly different than cataract surgery alone. Although traditional combined surgery involving trabeculectomy is performed less often, combined procedures involving minimally invasive glaucoma surgery are on the rise.

Which glaucoma procedure to combine with cataract extraction is dependent primarily on the severity of the glaucoma? As a general rule, I prefer combined phacoemulsification and trabeculectomy or implantation of the EX-PRESS Glaucoma Filtration Device (Alcon Laboratories) in patients with very advanced disease who are at high risk for severe functional impairment from glaucoma. Phacoemulsification combined with minimally invasive glaucoma surgery is most appropriate for mild to moderate disease, and cataract surgery alone may be the best option for visually significant cataract associated with ocular hypertension or easily controlled glaucoma.

Up to this point, we have been discussing a scenario in which an individual with glaucoma has a visually significant cataract requiring surgery. However, there are situations during which the glaucoma surgery is indicated, and the surgeon must decide how to manage the lens. In general, my indications for lens removal are more liberal in patients with pre-existing glaucoma. For example, I will remove a marginally significant cataract during a planned trabeculectomy, knowing that the cataract will likely progress following the glaucoma surgery. Likewise, if a patient needs lower IOP and has definite cataractous lens changes, I will discuss the option of early cataract surgery as an incremental step in the management of the glaucoma. When a patient has a cataract but is not experiencing symptoms, medications and laser trabeculoplasty are often used to buy time until symptoms for the cataract are more evident. The next section will briefly discuss the various forms of combined surgery in greater detail.

Combined Phacoemulsification and Guarded Filtration Surgery (Trabeculectomy and EX-PRESS Procedure)

Coincident phacoemulsification and trabeculectomy remain the most common combined glaucoma procedure for patients with severe glaucoma. Typically, phacoemulsification is performed in the standard fashion through a clear corneal incision, whereas the trabeculectomy is performed superiorly using standard techniques. Many glaucoma surgeons perform guarded filtration surgery utilizing the EX-PRESS Glaucoma Filtration Device beneath a scleral flap. Whether standard trabeculectomy or the EX-PRESS device is used, there is a definite trend toward fornix-based conjunctival flaps (Figure 4-1).[4] The use of adjunctive mitomycin-C has become standard protocol. The scleral flap is closed to avoid perioperative hypotony. Laser suture lysis or suture release is utilized to titrate IOP into the desired range. Although the efficacy of guarded filtration surgery is excellent, the added risk inherent to filtration blebs suggests that this procedure may be best reserved for patients with significant risk for severe functional impairment from glaucoma. Early to midterm postoperative results of trabeculectomy are excellent, but bleb survival remains vulnerable to the healing whims of the conjunctiva, often resulting in late failures. Although

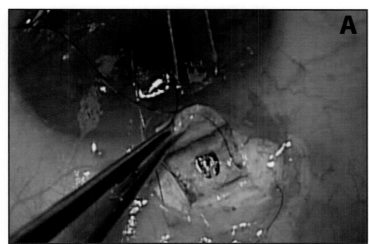

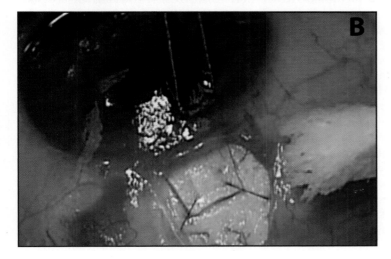

Figure 4-1. After completion of clear corneal phacoemulsification, the filtration surgery is performed superiorly. (A) Fornix-based conjunctival flap with EX-PRESS Implant in place. (B) Scleral flap sutures to titrate aqueous outflow.

antimetabolites, such as mitomycin-C, greatly enhance the success of trabeculectomy, the avascular or thinned conjunctiva is more prone to late bleb leaks, hypotony, and, perhaps most concerning, late bleb infection. Improved bleb morphology utilizing recent techniques, such as diffuse mitomycin-C exposure and fornix-based conjunctival incisions, have reduced the incidence of these serious complications.

Canaloplasty and Deep Sclerectomy

Viscocanalostomy and nonpenetrating deep sclerectomy were conceived with the goal of controlling IOP without the hazards of a filtration bleb, canaloplasty and viscocanalostomy, or creating a safer bleb. Stegmann et al[5] led a resurgence of interest in viscocanalostomy in the late 1990s. Although the Stegmann viscocanalostomy is truly "blebless," most versions of nonpenetrating deep sclerectomy still create a filtration bleb. Both procedures rely on the flow of aqueous through an exquisitely thin "trabeculo-Descemet" membrane. Such procedures are technically more difficult to perform and, like trabeculectomy, may be prone to late scarring. In addition, such procedures are "ab-externo," utilizing the superior conjunctiva and sclera. Accordingly, more traditional filtration surgery may be a less viable option in eyes that have undergone these procedures. These limitations have constrained the adoption of these procedures in the United States, although nonpenetrating glaucoma surgery remains popular in Europe. Despite limited adoption, nonpenetrating surgery is an acceptably safe and effective procedure to lower IOP and can be combined with phacoemulsification. Perhaps more importantly, with the renewed interest in procedures involving Schlemm's canal, these procedures have paved the way for more technologically sophisticated devices that bypass the trabecular meshwork and facilitate the flow of aqueous directly into the canal itself.

Ab-Interno Trabeculectomy and Trabecular Micro-Bypass Devices

Trabecular bypass stents represent the most recent effort toward blebless glaucoma surgery. Such procedures are based on the premise that the pathology in the physiological outflow system resides in the juxtacanalicular portion of the meshwork or within the inner wall itself. Outflow may be enhanced by ablating the inner wall with the Trabecome (NeoMedix Corporation)[6] or bypassing it with the proximal trabecular meshwork, facilitating the flow of aqueous into Schlemm's canal by providing a direct inlet into the canal (iStent Trabecular Micro-Bypass stent) or by direct communication and canal stenting (Hydrus; Ivantis Inc). Other devices, such as the SOLX Gold Shunt (SOLX Inc), the Glaukos Suprachoroidal Stent Model G-3 (Glaukos Corporation) and CyPass Micro-Stent (Transcend Medical Inc), divert aqueous into the suprachoroidal space. Excimer laser trabeculostomy utilizes the excimer laser to ablate trabecular tissue and provides direct communication of aqueous into Schlemm's canal.

With the exception of Trabectome and iStent, the other devices are investigational. The fact that the mentioned procedures can be readily performed coincidently with cataract surgery as part of a glaucoma-combined procedure suggests they may play an increasingly important role. The iStent was approved by the FDA in July 2012 and is indicated for use in early to moderate glaucoma. It is implanted as a combined procedure with cataract extraction. The iStent is implanted following completion of phacoemulsification and intraocular lens implantation. Knowledge of the angle anatomy and excellent intraoperative gonioscopy skills are essential for each of these procedures.

Although the concept of trabecular bypass is intriguing and promising, much work remains to be done. Some investigators have expressed concern over the lack of circumferential flow within Schlemm's canal. In other words, even if the trabecular meshwork is successfully bypassed with a stent, there is evidence to suggest that the outflow enhancement may be limited to several clock-hours surrounding the stent or perhaps the stent could miss the important collector channels completely. In this case, multiple stents or shunts may be needed to lower IOP adequately. Indeed, while the efficacy of a single iStent is modest, most surgeons believe that placing more than one stent, or ablating more of the meshwork in the case of ab-interno trabeculectomy, improves the IOP-reducing effect.

Endoscopic Cyclophotocoagulation

Endoscopic cyclophotocoagulation is yet another option for the coincident management of cataract and glaucoma. The procedure is performed through a clear corneal incision and is considered by many to be tailor-made as an adjunct to cataract surgery because access to the ciliary processes is greatly enhanced in pseudophakic eyes. Despite the lack of any prospective randomized trials, this technique has a loyal following of surgeons who perform this procedure for the management of milder forms of glaucoma to reduce the burden of medical therapy. Although many surgeons prefer to lower IOP by enhancing outflow, there is a definite role for endoscopic cyclophotocoagulation in the reduction of IOP in select patients.

Conclusion

The simultaneous presentation of cataract and glaucoma remains one of the most common comorbidities facing the anterior segment surgeon. The surgical options continue to evolve and improve. The management decisions should be individualized to both the patient and the surgeon to maximize outcomes and minimize risk. Ultimately, we are in a period of transition, and change may be the only constant as our medical and surgical options continue to improve.

References

1. Mansberger S, Gordon M, Jampel H, et al; Ocular Hypertension Treatment Study Group. Reduction in intraocular pressure after cataract extraction: the Ocular Hypertension Treatment Study. *Ophthalmology.* 2012;119(9):1826-1831.
2. Samuelson TW, Katz LJ, Wells JM, Duh YJ, Giamporcaro JE; US iStent Study Group. Randomized evaluation of the trabecular micro-bypass stent with phacoemulsification in patients with glaucoma and cataract. *Ophthalmology.* 2011;118(3):459-467.
3. Poley BJ, Lindstrom RL, Samuelson TW, Schulze R Jr. Intraocular pressure reduction after phacoemulsification with intraocular lens implantation in glaucomatous and nonglaucomatous eyes: evaluation of a causal relationship between the natural lens and open-angle glaucoma. *J Cataract Refract Surg.* 2009;35(11):1946-1955.
4. Maris P, Ishida K, Netland P. Comparison of trabeculectomy with EX-PRESS miniature glaucoma device implanted under scleral flap. *J Glaucoma.* 2007;16(1):14-19.
5. Stegmann R, Pienaar A, Miller D. Viscocanalostomy for open-angle glaucoma in black African patients. *J Cataract Refractive Surg.* 1999;25(3):316-322.
6. Francis BA, Minckler D, Dustin L, et al; Trabectome Study Group. Combined cataract extraction and trabeculotomy by the internal approach for coexisting cataract and open-angle glaucoma: initial results. *J Cataract Refract Surg.* 2008;34(7):1096-1103.

WHAT SHOULD I DO DIFFERENTLY IN PATIENTS AT HIGH RISK FOR RETINAL COMPLICATIONS?

Steve Charles, MD, FACS, FICS and
Eric J. Sigler, MD

The technical effort and time demands on the refractive cataract surgeon are enormous and have the potential of interfering with detailed preoperative assessment of the macula and peripheral retina. The retina can be visualized sufficiently in most cataract surgery patients in developed countries to enable a reasonable determination of the presence of most macular and retinal disorders. Spectral-domain optical coherence tomography (OCT) is far superior to time-domain OCT and enables the diagnosis of many macular disorders prior to cataract surgery. Clearly, the cataract surgeon should have second thoughts about implanting a multifocal intraocular lens in a patient with a macular disorder because of the potential reduction in contrast sensitivity.

Informed consent and exceeding or meeting patient expectations are crucial in the refractive cataract surgery setting. Diabetic macular edema, age-related macular degeneration (AMD), and high myopia all have the potential to affect outcomes and management strategies.

High Myopia

Myopia has not been shown to cause retinal detachment directly, but lattice-associated retinal holes are often coinherited with myopia. Myopia can be thought of as a proxy for lattice degeneration and retinal breaks. Greater axial length does not directly cause retinal detachment, but it should emphasize the need for careful preoperative peripheral retinal examination with the indirect ophthalmoscope, possibly by a retinal surgeon. Laser retinopexy of all holes or breaks in the lattice prior to cataract surgery is essential and relatively noncontroversial. Some retinal specialists treat only symptomatic retinal breaks, which I believe is overly conservative, especially in view of the extremely low complication rate of laser retinopexy if no retrobulbar block is performed. I recommend treating all retinal holes and breaks prior to cataract surgery or laser in situ keratomileusis surgery. History of retinal detachment in the fellow eye and family history of retinal detachment should increase awareness of the potential for retinal detachment after cataract surgery.

Myopic macular degeneration, like lattice degeneration, is not directly caused by greater axial length; however, myopic macular degeneration is often coinherited with high myopia. Myopic macular degeneration is somewhat similar to AMD in that it may have geographic atrophy or choroidal neovascular membranes that respond to intravitreal antivascular endothelial growth factor therapy. A very high myope with a normal-appearing macula is not at risk for myopic macular degeneration, whereas a patient with –5.00 diopters and lacquer cracks is at risk to develop geographic atrophy and choroidal neovascular membranes. Cystoid macular edema and inflammation are unrelated to myopic macular degeneration as well as to AMD, epimacular membranes, macular holes, and vitreomacular traction syndrome.

Diabetic Macular Edema

Cystoid macular edema after cataract surgery often is mistaken for worsening of diabetic macular edema; however, they often coexist or represent cystoid macular edema superimposed on diabetic macular edema. Both require treatment. The antivascular endothelial growth factor agent, ranibizumab, has been shown by a Diabeic Retinopathy Clinical Research Network randomized clinical trial[1] to be more effective than laser and much more effective than intravitreal steroids. In my opinion, intravitreal steroids are vastly overutilized in diabetic macular edema. Ranibizumab, potentially combined with PASCAL (patterned scanning laser; Topcon Medical Laser Systems)-style, short-duration, low-intensity, focal laser, is the safest, most effective management paradigm for diabetic macular edema. Topical nonsteroidal anti-inflamatory drugs (NSAIDS), such as nepafenac (Nevanac) or bromfenac ophthalmic solution (Bromday), for 6 to 8 weeks and difluprednate for 2 weeks are ideal for the treatment of cystoid macular edema (ie, Irvine-Gass syndrome) and may be used for several days preoperatively to reduce postsurgical inflammatory cystoid macular edema. For uncomplicated cataract extraction with an intact posterior capsule, extended postoperative NSAIDS are not required. Topical NSAIDS may be discontinued when iris inflammation (the anterior chamber cells) has subsided, usually within several days to weeks after surgery. Interestingly, Arevalo[2,3] has shown that intravitreal bevacizumab (Avastin) is effective in the treatment of cystoid macular edema in nondiabetic patients. Nepafenac or bromfenac may have some efficacy in diabetic macular edema, but topical steroids should not be used for DME because of the exceptionally long course of the disease.

Age-Related Macular Degeneration

Analysis of the Age-Related Eye Disease Study (AREDS) data[4] and additional reports[5] on AMD patients who underwent cataract surgery have demonstrated that cataract surgery does not affect AMD progression. A recent article that evaluated data from the Beaver Dam Eye Study suggested that 5-year follow-up of patients with cataract or cataract surgery had a somewhat higher incidence of late AMD.[6] In my opinion, that article should not alter the management of patients with a visually significant cataract. Precautions in patients with significant drusen or established drusen include instructing patients on use of the Amsler grid or digital self-monitoring application, smoking cessation, AREDS-identified antioxidants, and instructing staff that visual disturbances should be managed by prompt referral to a retina specialist.

As mentioned previously, spectral-domain, grey-scale OCT, such as SPECTRALIS (Heidelberg Engineering) or Cirrus (Carl Zeiss Meditec Inc), is far superior to time-domain

OCT, such as Stratus (Carl Zeiss Meditec Inc). Pseudocolor display of OCT images, thickness measurements, thickness maps, and 3-dimensional renderings often mask subtle subretinal fluid, resulting in a misdiagnosis of CME. There is no substitute for looking at all the B-scan slices of a spectral-domain, grey-scale OCT[7] to differentiate between epimacular membrane, macular schisis, vitreomacular traction syndrome, diabetic macular edema, cystoid macular edema, pigment epithelial detachment, and choroidal neovascular membranes. Some vitreoretinal experts incorrectly believe that vitreomacular traction syndrome can cause wet AMD; the reality is that both conditions are common and they often coexist. They both cause macular "elevation," AMD via subretinal or intraretinal fluid, and vitreomacular traction syndrome by mechanical means. Not all that is thick on OCT is edema; for example, foveal inversion after successful epimacular membrane surgery with internal limiting membrane peeling results in increased thickness, but it is not edema, it does not respond to steroids, and it will subside without treatment.

Conclusion

The cataract surgeon should be aware of special populations, including those with diabetic macular edema, AMD, and high myopia. Patients with high-risk features of their disease should be evaluated by a retinal specialist prior to cataract surgery. Prolonged use of topical NSAIDs and steroids is not necessary with routine cataract surgery, but it is helpful in patients with cystoid macular edema and diabetic macular edema.

References

1. Diabetic Retinopathy Clinical Research Network, Elman MJ, Qin H, et al. Intravitreal ranibizumab for diabetic macular edema with prompt versus deferred laser treatment: three-year randomized trial results. *Ophthalmology.* 2012;119(11):2312–2318.
2. Arevalo JF, Garcia-Amaris RA, Roca JA, et al; Pan-American Collaborative Retina Study Group. Primary intravitreal bevacizumab for the management of pseudophakic cystoid macular edema: pilot study of the Pan-American Collaborative Retina Study Group. *J Cataract Refract Surg.* 2007;33(12):2098-2105.
3. Arevalo JF, Maia M, Garcia-Amaris RA, et al; Pan-American Collaborative Retina Study Group. Intravitreal bevacizumab for refractory pseudophakic cystoid macular edema: the Pan-American Collaborative Retina Study Group results. *Ophthalmology.* 2009;116(8):1481-1487.
4. Chew EY, Sperduto RD, Milton RC, et al. Risk of advanced age-related macular degeneration after cataract surgery in the Age-Related Eye Disease Study: AREDS report 25. *Ophthalmology.* 2009;116(2):297-303.
5. Wang JJ, Fong CS, Rochtchina E, et al. Risk of age-related macular degeneration 3 years after cataract surgery: paired eye comparisons. *Ophthalmology.* 2012;119(11):2298-2303.
6. Klein BE, Howard KP, Lee KE, et al. The relationship of cataract and cataract extraction to age-related macular degeneration: the Beaver Dam Eye Study. *Ophthalmology.* 2012;119(8):1628-1633.
7. Brar M, Bartsch DU, Nigam N, et al. Colour versus grey-scale display of images on high-resolution spectral OCT. *Br J Ophthalmol.* 2009;93(5):597-602.

QUESTION

WHAT IS SPHERICAL ABERRATION, AND HOW DO I KNOW WHEN TO PUT IN A POSITIVE, NEGATIVE, OR NEUTRAL SPHERICAL ABERRATION INTRAOCULAR LENS?

Farrell C. Tyson, MD, FACS

Spherical aberration is an optical distortion when the peripheral light rays do not come into focus at the same focal point as central light rays. The patient usually perceives this as haloing of lights, especially in dim illumination when the pupil is dilated. Spherical aberration is labeled positive when the peripheral light rays come into focus in front of the central light rays. This is seen to the greatest effect in large myopic radial keratotomy and myopic laser in situ keratomileusis (LASIK) treatments. Negative spherical aberration is seen when the peripheral light rays come into focus behind the central light rays. This is most common in patients who have undergone hyperopic LASIK treatments.

In an ideal world, the optical system of an eye would have zero spherical aberration, with all light rays converging on one focal point. In reality, the human eye has a prolate cornea with different keratometric values between the central and peripheral cornea. A population distribution analysis of spherical aberration was performed on a predominately northern European patient base, which revealed the average amount of spherical aberration to be +0.27 μm[1]. A different study on Asian eyes found that the average amount of spherical aberration in this population to be +0.31 μm.[2] This information led lens manufactures to develop aspheric intraocular lens (IOL) designs to increase contrast sensitivity and decrease halos.

Choosing the Intraocular Lens

Initially, the standard IOL design consisted of a spherical optic that induced positive spherical aberration. These lenses, in average eyes, made the spherical aberration of the patient's optical system worse. Standard lenses still have an optimal benefit in patients with previous hyperopic LASIK or negative corneal asphericity.

Table 6-1

Spherical Aberration Profile of Different Intraocular Lenses

Manufacturer	Model	Asphericity
Abbott Medical Optics	Clariflex	Positive
Alcon Laboratories	SA60AT	Positive
Bausch & Lomb	LI61SE	Positive
Abbott Medical Optics	AR40e	Zero
Bausch & Lomb	LI61AO, Crystalens AO	Zero
STAAR Surgical	CC4204A, CQ2015A	−0.02 µm
Alcon Laboratories	Toric and ReSTOR Aspheric	−0.10 µm
Hoya Surgical Optics	iSymm	−0.18 µm
Alcon Laboratories	SN60WF	−0.17 to −0.20 µm
Abbott Medical Optics	TECNIS 1-piece, Toric, Multifocal	−0.27 µm

Over time, manufacturers started producing IOLs with varying amounts of spherical aberration correction from 0 to –0.27 µm (Table 6-1). This allows surgeons who are inherently limited to a theoretical accuracy of less than 0.25 diopters on IOL calculations to treat one more source of optical error, thus improving patient vision but also allowing happier patients who might still have residual refractive error.

The key to reducing spherical aberration in the patient's optical system is determining the patient's corneal spherical aberration preoperatively. Preoperatively, we are not interested in the patient's total spherical aberration, as the cataract will be removed, thus affecting total spherical aberration.

Several devices are now available that can obtain a patient's corneal spherical aberration, such as iTrace (Tracey Technologies), ARK-10000 (OPD-Scan; NIDEK Co Ltd). When the patient's corneal spherical abberation is known, an appropriate IOL can be selected to minimize the resultant total spherical aberration. In average-to-high amounts of positive spherical aberration, the TECNIS platform (Abbott Medical Optics Inc) reduces the most abberation and would be the most beneficial in centered, postmyopic LASIK ablation patients. On the other hand, no-to-small amounts of positive spherical aberration optimally would be treated with a Bausch & Lomb crystalens IOL AO platform or an Alcon aspheric IOL platform.

Spherical aberration reduction requires two things to be of benefit: good IOL centration and a pupil that is large enough. Spherical aberration is treated most effectively when the optics line up on the optical axis. This is the case in the majority of the time; however, in some scenarios, such as weak zonules, decentered ablation, or a large angle kappa, the IOL may not end up being centered on the optical axis. In these cases, a zero spherical aberration lens would be the optimal choice, as mild-to-moderate decentration does not affect these IOLs. Pupil size is important in determining the relative usefulness of aspheric optics versus symmetric optics. When the pupil is smaller than 3 mm, you effectively have a pinhole effect and peripheral light rays are rejected.[3] Therefore, in individuals with very small-pupils, aspheric IOLs have no advantage or disadvantage compared with standard IOLs. When contemplating monovision, neither design has a benefit on depth of focus at near visual acuity, as the pinhole effect is what drives the depth of focus. At intermediate and distance visual acuity, when the pupil will not be reflexively constricting the aspheric optics, monovision will allow for higher acuities and contrast sensitivity.

Multifocal IOLs, as a design, are able to obtain 2 focal points by splitting light into distance and near. This splitting of light is accomplished with a loss of contrast sensitivity. To overcome this inherent design limitation, the manufacturers have incorporated aspheric designs into their multifocal lenses. The different manufacturers have approached this with differing amounts of aspheric correction, which allows the surgeon to custom match the patient's corneal spherical aberration to the appropriate multifocal IOL. This helps to reduce perceived glare and halo, while improving the contrast sensitivity needed for improved reading vision.

Conclusion

It may seem a daunting task to treat not only refractive error but also spherical aberration. Yet, with the wide variety of spherical aberration correction amounts from the different manufacturers, we are now truly able to provide customized cataract surgery for our patients. This leads to happier patients and a growing practice.

References

1. Holladay JT, Piers PA, Koranyi G, van der Mooren M, Norrby NE. A new intraocular lens design to reduce spherical aberration of pseudophakic eyes. *J Refract Surg*. 2002;18(6):683-691.
2. Lim KL, Fam HB. Ethnic differences in higher-order aberrations: spherical aberration in the South East Asian Chinese eye. *J Cataract Refract Surg*. 2009;35(12):2114-2118.
3. Petermeier K, Frank C, Gekeler F, et al. Influence of the pupil size on visual quality and spherical aberration after implantation of the Tecnis 1-piece intraocular lens. *Br J Ophthalmol*. 2011;95(1):42-45.

My Patient Wants Enhanced Depth of Focus and Spectacle Independence. How Should I Decide Between Monovision or a Presbyopia-Correcting Intraocular Lens?

Sumitra Khandelwal, MD; David R. Hardten, MD; and Richard L. Lindstrom, MD

Patient expectations after cataract surgery are higher than ever, with many patients requesting to be spectacle-free. As a cataract surgeon, a strong understanding of the available intraocular lens (IOL) options aids in patient education and guidance. In addition, it is important to understand your patient's visual demands and expectations. A myopic patient who is used to taking off his or her glasses to read may not appreciate the reduced magnification that is experienced when using readers. In contrast, a previously hyperopic patient may have lower expectations of near vision, as these patients always use readers for near work. Understanding what lifestyle activities are important to the patient will help you to choose the most appropriate lens for your patient.

Available Lens Options

Monofocal Lens

Monofocal IOLs have one strong focus point. A balance exists between enhanced depth of focus and quality of vision, with the monofocal lens representing the least range of focus; however, spherical aberration may be customized to individual patients with some of the new lenses that are manufactured to specific spherical-aberration targets. Spherical aberration is now controlled in some lenses to impart negative (prolate modified) or neutral spherical aberrations, whereas other lenses are not specifically managed during manufacturing and have various levels of positive spherical aberration. Minimizing the total spherical aberration of the eye may be possible by choosing a lens to neutralize the spherical aberration of the patient's cornea.

A standard spherical monofocal IOL typically has positive spherical aberration. By using these standard lenses in patients who have corneas with negative spherical aberration, such as those with keratoconus or prior hyperopic refractive surgery, the spherical aberration of the eye may be less than using prolate-modified IOLs. In the majority of patients, the cornea has natural, positive spherical aberration, and a prolate-modified IOL may lead to fewer overall aberrations.

One implant tailored to have no lenticular spherical aberration is the SofPort AO (Bausch & Lomb Inc). Lenses manufactured with negative spherical aberration include the AcrySof SN60WF (Alcon Laboratories) and the TECNIS series, such as the Z9002, ZA9003, and ZCB00 (Abbott Medical Optics Inc). Negative spherical aberration lenses may be a good choice when the cornea has significant positive spherical aberration, such as a normal cornea or after myopic keratorefractive surgery.

MULTIFOCAL INTRAOCULAR LENS

Multifocal IOLs provide more than one focal plane, most by alternating zones of distant and near focus. Both distance and near uncorrected vision may be possible, also with improvement in intermediate uncorrected vision compared with a monofocal lens.[1] A loss of contrast sensitivity and a decrease in night vision quality may occur, and other coexisting ocular pathology may accentuate these side effects.

One class of multifocal IOL is the refractive group, with one example being the ReZoom IOL (Abbott Medical Optics Inc). ReZoom is a zonal aspheric multifocal lens that has 5 zones, alternating for distance and near. The refractive performance is pupil-size dependent, and, with bright light and small pupil size, the central zone is dominant for distance vision. In medium lighting, the more peripheral zones become available for near vision.

Another group of multifocal IOLs is the diffractive lens group such as the ReSTOR (Alcon Laboratories) and the TECNIS Multifocal (Abbott Medical Optics Inc). The TECNIS multifocal lens is an acrylic lens with an anterior prolate surface, which compensates for positive spherical aberration in the cornea, and a diffractive posterior surface. The diffractive rings for both distance and near are available in multiple lighting conditions, allowing less pupil-size dependence than the refractive category of multifocal IOLs.

The ReSTOR lens (Alcon Laboratories) is an acrylic lens with an anterior apodized diffractive optic and is manufactured with prolate spherical aberration. This lens is available in multiple add powers to tailor the near distance refractive target for patients.

ACCOMMODATING INTRAOCULAR LENS

Accommodating IOLs attempt to mimic the natural accommodation of the natural lens. It is still controversial whether this is the mechanism of range of focus by these lenses; yet, they appear to allow increased depth of focus. Night vision and contrast sensitivity may not be affected to the same degree with this category of lenses; yet, there are limits to the depth of focus achieved with these lenses. One example of lenses in this category available in the United States is the Crystalens (Bausch & Lomb Inc). The Crystalens is available in various optical zone sizes and aberration profiles.

TORIC INTRAOCULAR LENS

Toric IOLs are available for the correction of astigmatism at the time of surgery. Currently, they are only available as a monofocal IOL in the United States; however, multifocal toric IOLs may be available in the near future.

Methods of Intraocular Lens Use to Improve Spectacle Independence

Monovision

Pseudoaccommodative amplitude is approximately 2 diopters (D), allowing a patient who is targeted for –1.50 D to read as if wearing a +2.00 to +2.50 D addition lens. When one eye is targeted for distance and the other for near, enhanced depth of focus occurs binocularly.[2] Monovision creates anisometropia and may diminish stereopsis. Many patients tolerate monovision, but there are some that will not tolerate this anisometropia. A contact lens trial may help the decision; yet, when cataract is already present, assessment of the visual result after surgery is difficult. Patients who have previously worn monovision contact lenses and who are less tolerant of potential nighttime glare or halos and those who were previously myopic or postrefractive surgery often benefit the most from pseudophakic monovision.

Intermediate Vision

If intermediate vision is of the utmost importance to a particular patient, consider monofocal IOLs set for "mini-monovision," with the nondominant eye in the –1.00- to –1.50-D range for intermediate vision. A second option would be to use an accommodating IOL in 1 or both eyes, which is typically better at providing intermediate rather than near vision. It is important for the patient to understand that it is likely they will need to use reading glasses for near work or very fine print after receiving an accommodating IOL.

Near Vision

Multifocal lenses are typically the best option for patients who want to be spectacle-free for most scenarios. As previously mentioned, there are a number of different lens options; practically, these lenses are better at providing near and distance vision, with less power for intermediate vision. We tend to avoid these lenses in patients who are intolerant of potential decreased contrast vision or glare or halo, such as pilots or truck drivers, and those postrefractive surgery, as higher-order aberrations can diminish vision quality with a multifocal lens. Hyperopic patients tend to be the most enthusiastic with these lenses, as it provides near vision without correction, which these presbyopic hyperopic patients have never experienced.

Mixing Lenses

Mixing lenses is an option for some patients. We have found that we can get the advantages from 2 lens designs without significantly increasing downsides from each. For example, placing a multifocal IOL in the nondominant eye and an accommodating lens in the other dominant eye may be an option for improving intermediate vision.

Enhancements

Residual refractive error is a common reason for dissatisfaction following cataract surgery.[3] Accurate biometry is essential, and topography is useful when performing lens selection. If a refractive target is missed, keratorefractive enhancement may be utilized, waiting 2 to 3 months for the refractive error to stabilize. For large refractive surprises, IOL exchange can be considered, but is best done within the first 1 to 2 months after surgery due to capsule fibrosis.

Neuroadaptation

Neuroadaptation is an important concept with use of lenses dissimilar to the natural crystalline lens. Approximately 80% of patients adapt to complementary optics early, whereas 20% may take longer, ranging from a few months to 1 year or more. Patients continue to adapt for as long as 1 year, and waiting for neuroadaptation can provide long-term satisfactory results.

Conclusion

With several IOL options to choose from, surgeons should keep in mind the patient's daily activities, visual goals, and preoperative findings. In addition, detailed counseling is essential in the decision for IOL implantation.

References

1. Davis EA, Hardten DH, Lindstrom RL. *Presbyopic Lens Surgery: A Clinical Guide to Current Technology*. Thorofare, NJ: SLACK Incorporated; 2007.
2. Zhang F, Sugar A, Jacobsen G, Collins M. Visual function and patient satisfaction: comparison between bilateral diffractive multifocal intraocular lenses and monovision pseudophakia. *J Cataract Refract Surg*. 2011;37(3):446-453.
3. Hardten DR. Troubleshooting symptoms after refractive IOLs. In: Chang DF, ed. *Mastering the Art of Multifocal IOLs*. Thorofare, NJ: SLACK Incorporated; 2008.

How Do I Pick the Right Intraocular Lens Formula for My Patient With a Longer or Shorter Than Average Eye?

Robin R. Vann, MD

In the past 15 years, many innovations have greatly improved the efficiency, safety, and outcomes of cataract surgery. With the growth of refractive surgery and the introduction of premium intraocular lenses (IOLs), cataract surgeons are pressured to improve refractive accuracy.

Estimating Intraocular Lens Position

The axial length (AL) of most eyes (72%) falls within 22.0 and 24.5 mm.[1] In these eyes, the current third-generation formulas (SRK/T, Holladay 1, Hoffer Q) are able to determine the estimated IOL position accurately for a good refractive outcome. However, when we try to apply the same ELP predictions for the 28% of eyes that fall outside of this range, postoperative refraction predictions become less accurate. To improve our accuracy in these eyes, we have to approach the calculations differently (Figure 8-1).

In mild axial myopia, defined as eyes between 24.5 and 26 mm in length (15% of all eyes),[1] most formulas still perform well. Of the third-generation formulas, the Holladay 1 formula is very accurate in this range, with the SRK/T formula a close second. In moderate to extreme axial myopia (>26 mm; 7% of eyes),[1] posterior staphylomas are more common and make it difficult to determine accurate AL measurements using A-scan ultrasound biometry. For an accurate reading of the AL, A-scan biometry is dependent on having the ultrasound waves reflect back to the probe. Because staphylomatous eyes have an irregular posterior wall, it is common for ultrasonographers to misdirect the probe to improve the reflected wave spike, resulting in an inaccurate reading of the AL. Therefore, in these eyes, we should rely on optical biometry (IOLMaster; Carl Zeiss Meditec Inc, or LENSTAR LS 900; Haag-Streit) or B-scan–assisted AL measurements to determine the true AL.

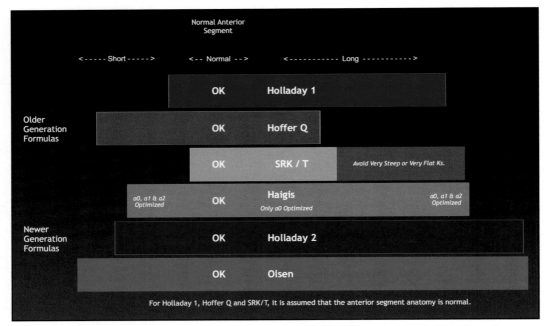

Figure 8-1. Guide for selecting the most accurate IOL formula based on axial length. Ks indicate keratometry readings; a0, a1, a2 are IOL constants. (Reprinted with permission of Warren E. Hill, MD.)

Despite using optical biometry to avoid the problem of posterior staphylomas, surgeons often find hyperopic refractive outcomes with third-generation formulas. Wang et al[2] believe that these highly myopic eyes have much more vitreous liquefaction, which changes the refractive index compared with normal eyes. Unfortunately, current optical biometers measure the whole eye using the same refractive index for all eyes and, as a result, provide an inaccurate AL measurement in eyes longer than 26 mm. Wang et al[2] have published a method of optimizing the AL measurement that can account for this hyperopic drift in these extremely myopic eyes:

Holladay 1: 2-center optimized AL = 0.8814 x IOLMaster AL + 2.8701

Haigis: 2-center optimized AL = 0.9621 x IOLMaster AL + 0.6763

SRK/T: 2-center optimized AL = 0.8981 x IOLMaster AL + 2.5637

Hoffer Q: 2-center optimized AL = 0.8776 x IOLMaster AL + 2.9269

In hyperopic eyes (AL <22 mm, 8% of all eyes),[1] accurate measurements and ELP predictions become even more important. The IOL power recommendations in these eyes tend to be much greater than in myopic eyes, so inaccuracies in ELP or IOL power recommendations can lead to greater prediction errors than in myopic eyes. Careful repetitive measurements are key in these eyes. In a study by MacLaren et al,[3] eyes measured with optical biometry and requiring IOL powers from 30.00 to 35.00 diopters had the smallest prediction errors when the Haigis, optimized on IOLMaster for one constant, or the Hoffer Q[4] formulas were used.

Conclusion

For anyone willing to take more eye measurements and invest in specialized IOL calculation software programs, newer formulas, such as the Holladay 2 and Olsen formulas, can provide more accurate predictions across the entire spectrum of ALs. The future of IOL calculation formulas is bright, with newer methods of modeling the eye for better ELP predictions coming in the next 2 to 3 years.

References

1. Fotedar R, Wang JJ, Burlutsky G, et al. Distribution of axial length and ocular biometry measured using partial coherence laser interferometry (IOL Master) in an older white population. *Ophthalmology.* 2010;117(3):417-423.
2. Wang L, Shirayama M, Ma XJ, Kohnen T, Koch DD. Optimizing intraocular lens power calculations in eyes with axial lengths above 25.0 mm. *J Cataract Refract Surg.* 2011;37(11):2018-2027.
3. MacLaren RE, Natkunarajah M, Riaz Y, et al. Biometry and formula accuracy with intraocular lenses used for cataract surgery in extreme hyperopia. *Am J Ophthalmol.* 2007;143(6):920-931.
4. Gavin EA, Hammond CJ. Intraocular lens power calculation in short eyes. *Eye (Lond).* 2008;22(7):935-938.

HOW DO I ADDRESS INTRAOCULAR LENS CALCULATIONS AND SELECTIONS IN THE POSTKERATOREFRACTIVE PATIENT?

Warren E. Hill, MD, FACS

Since the introduction of radial keratotomy in the United States in 1978, a conservative estimate is that close to 40 million eyes throughout the world have undergone some form of keratorefractive surgery. A predictable consequence of such wide acceptance of this strategy for the reduction of refractive errors for more than 3 decades is that these patients are now aging and undergoing cataract surgery in ever-increasing numbers.

Consequences of Prior Keratorefractive Surgery

In the beginning, no one imagined that several unanticipated consequences would follow keratorefractive surgery. These include an inability to accurately measure the central corneal power with standard equipment, intraocular lens (IOL) power calculation inaccuracies that require special modifications, and the inducement of higher-order aberrations.

Underappreciated is the fact that the presence of multiple, elevated higher-order aberrations has the potential both to reduce visual quality at larger pupil sizes and limit the success of IOL options offered with cataract surgery.

Physicians who routinely perform lens-based surgery for patients who have undergone prior keratorefractive surgery are keenly aware that these individuals are both emotionally and financially invested in a specific refractive outcome. It is not without some irony that the very procedure initially used to reduce dependence on spectacles may, much later, limit or even preclude spectacle independence.

Eyes with prior keratorefractive surgery can be divided into 3 basic categories: radial keratotomy (RK), hyperopic laser in situ keratomileusis (LASIK) or photorefractive keratotomy (PRK), and myopic LASIK/PRK. Selecting the correct IOL in these situations also has 3 basic components: the proper estimation of central corneal power, the use of a specific and specially modified

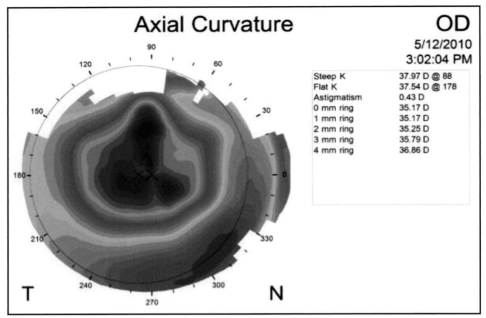

Figure 9-1. Zeiss ATLAS 9000 topographer axial curvature map of an eye with prior 8 incision radial keratotomy. Such eyes are often multifocal and frequently show an across-the-board increase in higher-order aberrations, such as positive spherical aberration and coma, with a corresponding loss in contrast sensitivity at larger pupil sizes.

IOL power calculation methodology, and the selection of the most appropriate IOL, with the type and amount of spherical aberration being significant. The approach to various combinations of incisional and ablative forms of keratorefractive surgery, such as RK plus LASIK is beyond the scope of this chapter.

Radial Keratotomy

Radial keratotomy can be approached in a relatively straightforward manner. Methods for the estimation of central corneal power that have been useful are as follows: the average of the 1.0-, 2.0-, 3.0-, and 4.0-mm annular (ring) power values of the Zeiss ATLAS corneal topographer[1] (Carl Zeiss Meditec Inc; Figure 9-1); the adjusted effective refractive power (EffRPadj) from the Holladay Diagnostic Summary of the EyeSys Corneal Analysis System (EyeSys Vision Inc); and the Pentacam Power Distribution Sagittal Power (OCULUS Inc) mean keratometry value for a 4.0-mm zone, centered on the pupil (Figure 9-2).[2-6]

For most theoretical formulas, the mathematical artifact produced by a nonphysiologic flat central cornea also must be addressed. Without the separation of contemporary measurements from the central corneal power used to estimate the effective lens position, formulas may assume that the IOL will be sitting in a more anterior position, resulting in less IOL power and unanticipated hyperopia. This effective lens-position correction is typically carried out by applying an Aramberri Double-K method correction[7] or by applying a similar built-in feature of the Holladay 2 formula, which is contained within the Holladay IOL Consultant Software (Holladay Consulting).[8]

Eyes with prior RK generally have an elevation of multiple higher-order aberrations, with spherical aberration and coma often dominating the aberration profile. Although it is not currently

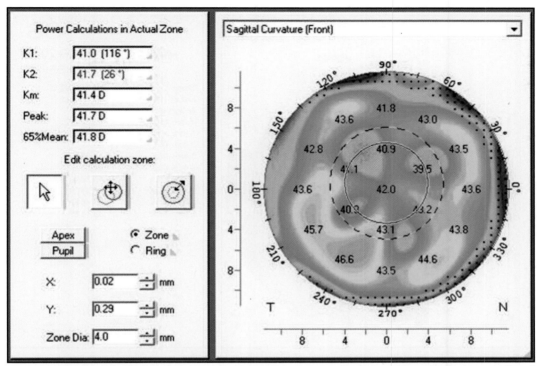

Figure 9-2. Power Distribution feature of the OCULUS Pentacam, displaying the sagittal curvature (front) mean keratometry value for a 4.0-mm zone, centered on the pupil. When used in conjunction with the Double-K method corrected theoretical formula and a RK-specific correction algorithm, this method has an accuracy similar to the Zeiss ATLAS topographer. This calculation method is available on the American Society of Cataract and Refractive Surgery's Web site.[1]

possible to correct all of the spherical aberrations with an IOL, it is possible to offset a portion. For this, the TECNIS IOL (Abbott Medical Optics Inc), with −0.275 μm of negative spherical aberration, or the AcrySof SN60WF IQ lens (Alcon Laboratories), with −0.200 μm of negative spherical aberration, can be useful choices. If possible, the surgeon should measure the anterior corneal spherical aberration prior to selecting the most appropriate IOL. The main objective is that the selected IOL should not increase the spherical aberration.

Multiple steep and flat meridians often preclude using a toric IOL in a predictable manner, and the loss of contrast due to higher-order aberrations generally make diffractive optics IOLs problematic.

Hyperopic Laser in Situ Keratomileusis

Eyes that have undergone prior hyperopic LASIK and PRK have some calculation similarities with prior RK. This is something of a paradox, as the first method is hyperopic ablative and the second is incisional myopic. Nonetheless, both methods result in an increase in the corneal Gullstrand ratio.

If the amount of hyperopic LASIK is less than +4.00 diopters, the average of the 1-, 2-, and 3-mm annular (ring) power values from the Zeiss ATLAS topographer or the EffRPadj from the Holladay Diagnostic Summary of the EyeSys Corneal Analysis System can be used to estimate

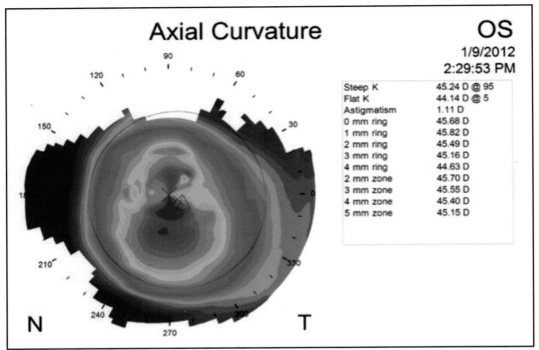

Figure 9-3. Zeiss ATLAS 9000 topographer axial curvature map of an eye with prior hyperopic LASIK. The central steepening of these corneas reduces the naturally occurring positive spherical aberration of the cornea. Following large amounts of hyperopic LASIK, the corneal spherical aberration value may shift negative.

the central corneal power. For higher powers, Wang et al[9] has shown that an additional correction may be needed. The hyperopic version of the Haigis-L[10], Masket[11], Shammas,[12] and modified Masket[13] formulas also have been shown to be useful. The Haigis-L formula[10] is especially useful when there is no prior refractive data or when some amount of regression has occurred.

Again, if using a theoretical formula, an Aramberri Double-K method correction should be carried out, or the Holladay 2 formula should be used, so that the IOL power calculation formula does not incorrectly estimate the effective lens position. As the Haigis formula does not tie the effective lens position calculation to the central corneal power, Haigis-L and Shammas are the exceptions because these formulas do not require a Double-K correction.

Eyes with prior hyperopic LASIK typically show a reduction in the naturally occurring anterior corneal spherical aberration because the central cornea has been steepened (Figure 9-3). If possible, an anterior corneal spherical aberration value should be obtained prior to deciding which IOL to use. If this value is low, then an aberration-neutral aspheric IOL, such as the Bausch & Lomb LI61AO, would be a reasonable choice. If the spherical aberration value has shifted negative, then a conventional spherical IOL, such as the AcrySof SN60AT (Alcon Laboratories) is preferred. Because the center of the cornea is often converted to a broad steep zone, the use of toric or multifocal IOLs may be problematic and generally are approached with caution.

IOL Powers Calculated Using Double-K Holladay 1 Formula Except Haigis-L and Shammas Method

Using Pre-LASIK/PRK Ks + ΔMR		Using ΔMR		Using no prior data	
		Adjusted EffRP	19.02		
		Adjusted Atlas 0-3	19.02	Wang-Koch-Maloney	18.90
Clinical History	19.65			Shammas Method	18.91
Feiz-Mannis	19.90	Masket Formula	18.36	Haigis-L	18.93
Corneal Bypass	19.79	Modified-Masket	18.97	Galilei	18.44
		Adjusted ACCP/ACP/APP	18.23		

Average IOL Power:	19.01	
Min:	18.23	
Max:	19.90	

Figure 9-4. The online postkeratorefractive surgery IOL power calculator of the American Society of Cataract and Refractive Surgery.[1] The surgeon enters data from instruments that are available, and a corresponding IOL power will be calculated. Abbreviation: MR, manifest refraction.

Myopic Laser in Situ Keratomileusis

Selecting the correct IOL for eyes that have undergone prior myopic LASIK can be the most challenging of the 3 common forms of keratorefractive surgery. This is because the central corneal power is reduced by the ablation of tissue.

For the calculation of IOL power after myopic LASIK, a wide range of methods have been proposed, all of which have limited accuracy. Some derive a set of keratometry values (Ks) from purely historical information, some modify measured Ks or a calculated IOL power based on the change in manifest refraction, and some base the calculation of IOL power solely on contemporary measurements.[1] Popular calculation methodologies are arranged in this way on the American Society of Cataract and Refractive Surgery's online Post Keratorefractive IOL Calculator[1] (Figure 9-4).

Following myopic LASIK, purely historical methods generally have the lowest overall accuracy. Of the methods that employ commonly used instrumentation, better accuracy is obtained with the Masket, modified Masket, myopic Haigis-L, and Shammas methods.[14] Eyes with prior myopic LASIK show an increase in the naturally occurring positive spherical aberration due to central corneal flattening (Figure 9-5). In the United States, the Alcon AcrySof SN60WF IQ and the Abbott Medical Optics TECNIS monofocal IOLs are widely used after myopic LASIK.

Conclusion

Patients undergoing phacoemulsification with IOL implantation following all forms of keratorefractive surgery will continue to be a challenge until a completely reliable method for calculating IOL power for each type of refractive surgery has been firmly established.

References

1. Hill W, Wang L, Koch DD. American Society of Cataract and Refractive Surgery post keratorefractive IOL calculator. Version 4.4. http://www.ascrs.org. Accessed September 10, 2012.

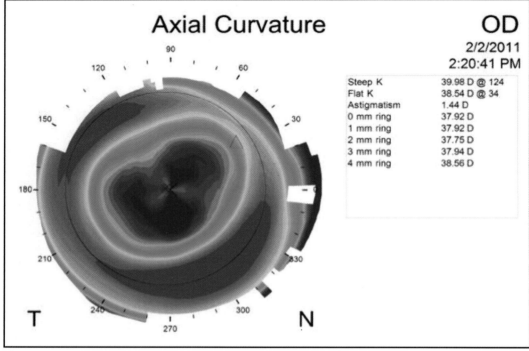

Figure 9-5. Zeiss ATLAS 9000 topographer axial curvature map of an eye with prior myopic LASIK. The central flattening of such corneas typically induces additional positive spherical aberration.

2. Hill WE. IOL calculations after refractive surgery. *Cataract and Refractive Surgery Today.* June 2012. http://www.bmctoday.net/crstoday/2012/06/article.asp?f=iol-calculations-after-refractive-surgery. Accessed June 13, 2013.

3. Fang JP, Hill W, Wang L, Chang V, Koch DD. Advanced intraocular lens power calculations. In: Kohnen T, Koch DD, eds. *Essentials in Ophthalmology: Cataract and Refractive Surgery.* 2nd ed. Berlin, Germany: Springer-Verlag; 2006:31-46.

4. Hill WE. IOL calculations after refractive surgery. *Advanced Ocular Care.* 2011;Nov/Dec:17-19.

5. Hill WE. IOLs and prior radial keratotomy: challenges for the cataract surgeon. Paper presented at: Annual Meeting of the American Society of Cataract and Refractive Surgery; April 2012; Chicago, IL.

6. Potvin R, Hill W. New algorithm for post-RK intraocular lens power calculations based on rotating scheimpflug camera data. *J Cataract Refract Surg.* 2013;39(3):358-365.

7. Aramberri J. Intraocular lens power calculation after corneal refractive surgery: double K method. *J Cataract Refract Surg.* 2003;29(11):2063-2068.

8. Koch D, Wang L. Calculating IOL power in eyes that have had refractive surgery. *J Cataract Refract Surg.* 2003;29(11):2039-2042.

9. Wang L, Jackson DW, Koch DD. Methods of estimating corneal refractive power after hyperopic laser in situ keratomileusis. *J Cataract Refract Surg.* 2002;28(6):954-961.

10. Haigis W. The Haigis-L Formula. Paper presented at: the European Society of Cataract and Refractive Surgeons meeting; September 2008; Berlin, Germany.

11. Masket S, Masket SE. Simple regression formula for intraocular lens power adjustment in eyes requiring cataract surgery after excimer laser photoablation. *J Cataract Refract Surg.* 2006;32(3):430-434.

12. Shammas HJ, Shammas MC, Hill WE. Intraocular lens power calculation in eye with previous hyperopic laser in situ keratomileusis. *J Cataract Refract Surg.* 2013;39(5):739-744.

13. Hill WE. Modification of the Masket regression formula. Paper presented at: Annual Meeting of the American Society of Cataract and Refractive Surgery; March 2006; San Francisco, CA.

14. Wang L, Hill WE, Koch DD. Evaluation of IOL power prediction methods using the ASCRS Post-Keratorefractive Intraocular Lens Power Calculator. *J Cataract Refract Surg.* 2010;36(9):1466-1473.

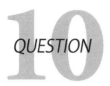

My Cataract Patient Has a Pterygium in the Operative Eye. How Do I Know if it Has an Impact on My Intraocular Lens Calculations? If So, What Should I Do?

Mahshad Darvish, MD and
Edward Holland, MD

Pterygia are fibrovascular growths of connective tissue that extend from the bulbar conjunctiva onto the cornea. They are associated with chronic exposure to sunlight, specifically ultraviolet type B radiation. Pterygia are most commonly found in the "pterygium belt," a region straddling the earth's equator; yet, with the increasing mobility of the global populace, they are becoming ubiquitous and a relevant issue for all ophthalmologists.

Evaluating a Patient With a Pterygium

Pterygia typically induce asymmetric, with-the-rule astigmatism in the axis of the advancing lesion.[1] When evaluating a patient with a pterygium and cataract, one must assess what is causing the decrease in vision. The visual disturbance could be a result of the pterygium alone, the cataract alone, or a combination of the two. As cataract surgery progresses toward better and better refractive outcomes, ophthalmologists cannot ignore the potentially confounding effects of pterygia. This is especially important when considering toric, accommodating, or multifocal intraocular lenses.

The first step in determining the importance of a pterygium is by history. It is important to determine if the patient complains of ocular surface irritation. An inflamed pterygium can reduce patient satisfaction after an uncomplicated cataract surgery. Next, a careful slit-lamp examination of the lesion should be performed. The pterygium should be evaluated for inflammation, proximity to the visual axis, and recent growth.

The size of the lesion and its distance from the visual axis should be noted. It has been shown that larger lesions that encroach to within 3 mm from the visual axis produce increasing amounts of induced astigmatism.[2] Two mechanisms have been proposed for this refractive effect: (1) pooling of the tear film at the leading edge of the pterygium and (2) mechanical traction placed on the cornea by the lesion. Such large pterygia produce increasingly irregular and asymmetric astigmatism that can interfere with accurate keratometry readings. Large pterygia can also inhibit docking with some femtosecond lasers used in cataract surgery.

In addition to a pterygium's size, its growth and stability should also be ascertained. In the absence of documented growth, the patient should be questioned to see if he or she has noted a change in the size of the lesion. Also, one should examine the patient's refractive stability. If the patient states that the pterygium has been the same size for many years and their manifest refraction has not changed significantly over the past 5 years, it is likely safe to proceed with the cataract surgery, provided good measurements can be obtained. Conversely, if the magnitude and axis of the patient's astigmatism have changed recently, or if he or she notes that the pterygium has grown, then excision is recommended prior to cataract surgery.

Patients with large amounts of astigmatism and a concurrent pterygium should be approached with a high level of caution. Even if the pterygium is stable, it is recommended that it be excised. This approach will allow for the optimum management of the astigmatism, ensured stability, and ultimately the best refractive outcomes.

Removal of pterygia has been shown to significantly reduce the astigmatism caused by moderate to large lesions as early as 1 month after surgery. This reduction in astigmatism is accompanied by improvements in the corneal surface and increased symmetry on topography.

Simultaneous excision of the pterygium and cataract surgery is not recommended, as refractive outcomes cannot be predicted accurately. Instead, it is recommended that a patient be monitored for stability on both topography and keratometry after excisional surgery before proceeding with cataract surgery.

Options

If the decision is made to remove the pterygium, several options are available. It is strongly recommended to combine the pterygium excision with an adjunct measure to minimize recurrence. Simple excisions leaving bare sclera have been found to have an unacceptably high recurrence rate, ranging from 30% to 80%.[3]

The procedure of choice is an excision combined with a conjunctival autograft. This technique has a significantly lower recurrence rate (2% to 5%) than a simple excision alone and avoids the potentially sight-threatening complications associated with medical adjuvants such as mitomycin-C (Mitozytrex or Mutamycin) and beta irradiation. Fibrin glue can be used to enhance the results of this procedure by reducing the recurrence rate, enhancing patient comfort, and decreasing operative times.

Amniotic membrane transplantation is an alternative adjunct procedure that is particularly useful in cases where large autografts are needed. However, it has not been shown to be superior to conjunctival autografts. In fact, 2 prospective studies, one randomized and one nonrandomized, found an unacceptably high recurrence rate with amniotic membrane transplants when compared with conjunctival autografts.[3]

Conclusion

In the era of refractive cataract surgery and increased global mobility, the importance of pterygium management cannot be overstated, nor can its relevance to all ophthalmologists, regardless of their geographic location. An aggressive approach is advocated. If there is any concern about a pterygium, it should be excised before the cataract surgery, and the patient should be followed by

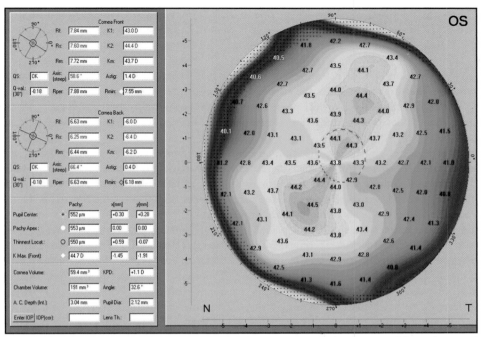

Figure 11-1. Corneal topography reveals regular astigmatism that is treatable with paired peripheral corneal-relaxing incisions that are each 1.4 clock-hours in length, centered on the steep meridian.

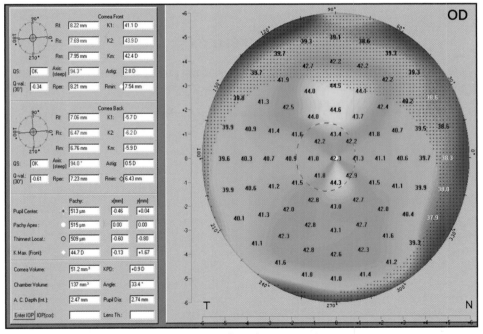

Figure 11-2. Topography measures 2.80 D of regular astigmatism.

and aspheric SN6AT lens models are available in 0.75 D increments. Cylinder power ranges from 1.50 to 6.00 D in the IOL plane, correcting 1.03 to 4.11 D astigmatism at the corneal plane. An aspheric IOL is recommended for eyes with normal, prolate corneas and positive spherical aberration.

Both the Alcon and STAAR Surgical online toric IOL calculators utilize vector analysis. Input required from the surgeon includes the axis and surgically induced astigmatism of the phacoemulsification incision, the IOL spherical power, and corneal topographic cylinder. The result identifies the IOL cylinder power, desired axis of implantation, and anticipated residual astigmatism (Figure 11-3).

For either IOL design, the implantation technique is the same. With the patient sitting upright, a reference mark is made at the limbus. We prefer a single mark at 6 o'clock. Other surgeons prefer paired marks at 3 o'clock and 9 o'clock, corresponding to the 180-degree meridian. Under the operating microscope, a corneal gauge guides the placement of marks on the desired IOL implantation axis, utilizing the prior limbal marks for reference.

After cataract extraction, the IOL is placed in the capsular bag and rotated to the marked corneal axis. Meticulous viscoelastic removal from the capsular bag is critical to minimize the chance of early postoperative IOL rotation. One must be careful to avoid unwanted movement and rotation of the IOL during viscoelastic aspiration. Small rotational adjustments are made to align the toric IOL marks on the desired axis before the incision is sealed.

For patients with >4.00-D corneal cylinder, a combination of toric IOL and PCRIs can be considered. We do not recommend paired PCRIs to treat >3.00-D cylinder, as this risks possible corneal instability and dry eye complications. For symptomatic residual astigmatism after cataract surgery, enhancement laser refractive surgery can be considered. In summary, surgeons have a variety of effective options to improve patients' visual function and satisfaction following cataract surgery.

References

1. Amesbury EC, Miller KM. Long-term clinical outcome after ReSTOR SA60D3 intraocular lens implantation. Paper presented at: American Society of Cataract and Refractive Surgery Symposium on Cataract, IOL, and Refractive Surgery; April 2010; Boston, MA.
2. Hill W. Expected effects of surgically induced astigmatism on AcrySof toric intraocular lens results. *J Cataract Refract Surg.* 2008;34(3):364-367.

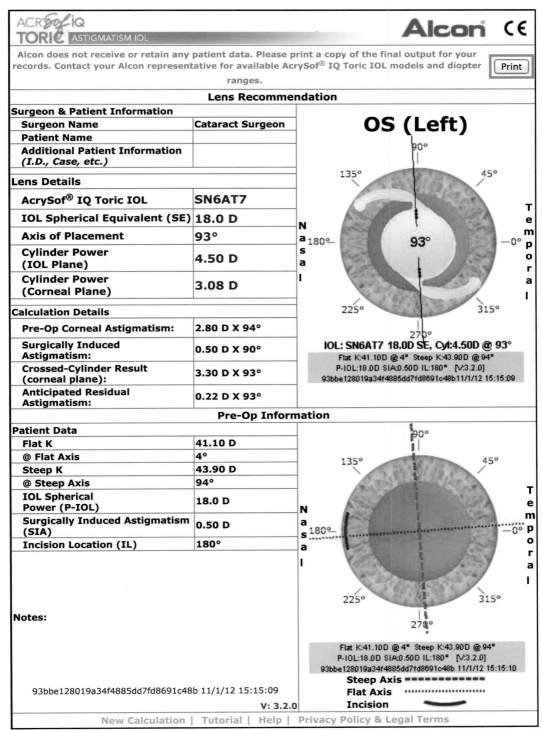

Figure 11-3. Sample toric IOL calculation for the eye in Figure 11-2. The Alcon SN6AT7, implanted through a temporal phacoemulsification incision, will result in approximately 0.20 D residual astigmatism. K indicates keratometry values. (Reproduced with permission of Alcon Laboratories.)

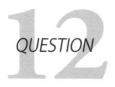
MY ASTIGMATIC KERATOTOMY RESULTS ARE UNPREDICTABLE. HOW CAN I IMPROVE THEM?

R. Bruce Wallace III, MD

Limbal-relaxing incisions (LRIs) are probably the friendliest and most cost-effective refractive procedures we can offer our patients. There is no expensive laser involved, no central corneal or intraocular trauma, and perforations are rare in healthy corneas. So, why is it that many cataract surgeons are not yet using LRIs? Some of us are not convinced that they are reliable, especially if, after purchasing the special instruments, the initial results were disappointing. For many, the awkwardness of incisional corneal surgery, along with an uncomfortable change in routine for surgeon and staff, has placed LRIs in a negative light. Yet, judging by the swell in attendance at teaching events like Skip Nichamin's LRI wet labs at the last few American Academy of Ophthalmology and American Society of Cataract and Refractive Surgeons meetings, LRIs are growing rapidly in popularity.

We owe a great deal of thanks to early pioneers who promoted the benefits of combining astigmatic keratotomy with cataract surgery many years ago. A partial list would include Drs. Gills, Hollis, Osher, Maloney, Shepherd, Koch, Thornton, Gayton, Davison, and Lindstrom. Robert Osher, MD, has advocated peripheral relaxing keratotomy at the time of cataract surgery since 1983,[1] having learned the principles of the technique from George Tate, MD.

I have had the pleasure of teaching LRI techniques with Drs. Nichamin, Maloney, Dillman, and many others for more than 20 years. During these training sessions, I have learned the steps necessary to convince cataract surgeons that LRIs can be an important part of refractive cataract surgery. Before a cataract surgeon transitions to the routine use of LRIs, he or she must understand the benefits, be confident in the "system" of treatment, and be confident with his or her technique.

Treatment Systems

A systematic approach to LRI use improves results. Drs. Gills, Lindstrom, Nichamin, and I have developed a number of LRI nomograms. I first used Nichamin's excellent nomogram and then modified it to slant more toward one incision for lower levels of cylinder (Tables 12-1 and 12-2). Because we make our incisions so far in the corneal periphery, paired incisions were found not to be as important for postoperative corneal regularity as traditional astigmatic keratotomy made at the 6-to 7-mm optical zone. An advantage of the Nichamin nomograms and their modification is that treatment is planned in degrees of arc rather than cord length. Degree measurements are universally more accurate because corneal diameters vary and because we make arcs, not straight-line incisions.

For lower levels of astigmatism (<2.00 diopters [D]), selecting the axis of cylinder can be challenging.[2] I look at all axis measurements but usually select ones from computerized corneal topography. Sometimes, especially with smaller cylinder corrections, there is poor correlation of the axis as determined by refraction, keratometry (K) readings, and topography. Many times, when I encounter this situation with first eyes for cataract surgery, I will postpone the LRI and measure the cylinder postoperatively. If there is visually disturbing postoperative astigmatism, I will perform LRIs centered on the axis of the postoperative refraction the same day the patient returns for cataract surgery in the fellow eye. Residual astigmatism in the first eye also alerts me to consider an LRI in the second eye.

Questions arise concerning intraocular lens (IOL) power modifications with LRIs. With low to moderate levels of cylinder (0.50 to 2.75 D), corneal "coupling" equalizes the central corneal power so there is less chance the IOL power selection will be inaccurate. Longer LRI incisions for higher cylinder (>3.00 D) may create a radial keratotomy-like flattening effect and produce unwanted postoperative hyperopia. Increasing the IOL power by 0.50 to 1.00 D may be necessary in these cases.

Instrumentation

Simplification of instruments and techniques improves efficiency and comfort with the procedure. There are many excellent LRI instrument sets available from Mastel Precision; Rhein Medical Inc; Katena Products Inc; ASICO; and others. I designed the Wallace LRI Kit with Bausch & Lomb's Storz Ophthalmic Instruments. This kit includes a pre-set, single foot plate, trifacet diamond knife (600 µm); a Mendez axis marker; and a −0.12-caliber forceps.

The trifacet diamond is less likely to chip. The Mendez marker has numbers on the dial to help guide the surgeon to the proper axis mark. This orientation guide is valuable because the biggest fear, besides a perforation, is placing the incision in the wrong axis. All of these instruments are made of titanium to increase longevity.

Patient Counseling

Similar to preoperative discussion of the new refractive IOLs, informing patients about the option of surgical treatment for astigmatism has become commonplace in many cataract practices. We start by describing the optical disadvantages of astigmatism and the relative effectiveness and low risk surrounding LRIs. In the United States, when charging Medicare patients for an additional out-of-pocket fee for LRIs, an advanced beneficiary notice should be filed.

Table 12-1
The "NAPA" Nomogram

Pachymetry-Adjusted Intralimbal Arcuate Astigmatic Nomogram With-the-Rule (Steep Axis 45 degrees to 145 degrees)

Preoperative	Paired Incisions in Degrees of Arc			
Cylinder (Diopters)	20 to 30 years old	31 to 40 years old	41 to 50 years old	51 to 60 years old
0.75	40	35	35	30
1.00	45	40	40	35
1.25	55	50	45	40
1.50	60	55	50	45
1.75	65	60	55	50
2.00	70	65	60	55
2.25	75	70	65	60
2.50	80	75	70	65
2.75	85	80	75	70
3.00	90	90	85	80

Against-the-Rule (Steep Axis 0 degrees to 40 degrees/140 degrees to 180 degrees)

Preoperative	Paired Incisions in Degrees of Arc			
Cylinder (Diopters)	20 to 30 years old	31 to 40 years old	41 to 50 years old	51 to 60 years old
0.75	45	40	40	35
1.00	50	45	45	40
1.25	55	55	50	45
1.50	60	60	55	50
1.75	65	65	60	55
2.00	70	70	65	60
2.25	75	75	70	65
2.50	80	80	75	70
2.75	85	85	80	75
3.00	90	90	85	80

When placing intralimbal-relaxing incisions following or concomitant with radial-relaxing incisions, total arc length is decreased by 50%.

Abbreviation: NAPA, Nichamin Age & Pachymetry-Adjusted Intralimbal Arcuate Astigmatic.

Created by and used with permission of Louis D. "Skip" Nichamin, MD of Laurel Eye Clinic, Brookville, Pennsylvania.

Table 12-2
Wallace Nomogram

Instruments
- Diamond knife: Trifacet 600 µm preset depth, single foot plate
- Marker: Mendez axis ring
- Forceps: 0.12 caliber

Procedure
- Place axis ring around limbus.
- Mark axis with forceps.
- Mark limits of intended incision(s) with forceps.
- Remove axis ring.
- Dry marks with cellulose sponge.
- Fixate globe with forceps.
- Perform incision(s), direct toward fixation.

Nomogram
Assuming all cataract incisions are performed temporally and are relatively astigmatical neutral:

For With-the-Rule and Oblique Astigmatism					
Astigmatism (in diopters)	*40 to 50 years old*	*50 to 60 years old*	*60 to 70 years old*	*70 to 80 years old*	*80+ years old*
1.00 to 1.50	60 degrees[1]	50 degrees[1]	50 degrees[1]	40 degrees[1]	30 degrees[1]
1.50 to 2.00	70 degrees[1]	70 degrees[1]	70 degrees[1]	60 degrees[1]	60 degrees[1]
2.00 to 2.50	60 degrees[2]	60 degrees[2]	60 degrees[2]	70 degrees[1]	70 degrees[1]
2.50 to 3.00	70 degrees[2]	70 degrees[2]	70 degrees[2]	60 degrees[2]	60 degrees[2]
3.00 to 4.00	80 degrees[2]	80 degrees[2]	80 degrees[2]	70 degrees[2]	70 degrees[2]
For Against-the-Rule Astigmatism					
Astigmatism (in diopters)	*40 to 50 years old*	*50 to 60 years old*	*60 to 70 years old*	*70 to 80 years old*	*80+ years old*
1.00 to 1.50	60 degrees[1]	50 degrees[1]	40 degrees[1]	40 degrees[1]	30 degrees[1]
1.50 to 2.00	70 degrees[1]	60 degrees[1]	60 degrees[1]	60 degrees[1]	40 degrees[1]
2.00 to 2.50	60 degrees[2]	80 degrees[1]	80 degrees[1]	70 degrees[1]	60 degrees[1]
2.50 to 3.00	70 degrees[2]	70 degrees[2]	70 degrees[2]	60 degrees[2]	60 degrees[2]
3.00 to 4.00	80 degrees[2]	80 degrees[2]	80 degrees[2]	70 degrees[2]	70 degrees[2]

[1] denotes 1 incision

[2] denotes 2 incisions

When using nomogram, if age/astigmatism at dividing point:
- Choose the shortest incision length
- Choose 1 incision over 2 incisions

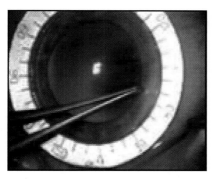

Figure 12-1. Marking the astigmatic axis with a Mendez ring.

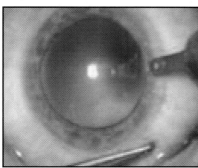

Figure 12-2. Limbal-relaxing incision placed 1.0 to 1.5 mm from the surgical limbus.

Technique

A surgeon's LRI technique will vary, depending on the instruments used for the procedure. The routine I use with the Duckworth & Kent instruments is as follows:

- Make the LRIs before making the phaco incision, but after wetting the cornea.
- Mark the axis (Mendez ring and 0.12 forceps).
- Mark the incision borders (Mendez ring and 0.12 forceps).
- Fixate the globe (0.12 forceps).
- Advance the knife toward fixation (usually toward the surgeon).

Try to insert the knife into the peripheral corneal dome (approximately 1.5 mm from the limbus) as perpendicular as possible (Figures 12-1 and 12-2). Maintain this blade orientation and, with moderate pressure, complete the LRI by "connecting the dots" on the cornea and twirling the knife handle to make an arcuate incision using the limbus as a template.

Postoperative Care

For many years, we added a nonsteroidal anti-inflammatory drug (NSAID) to our postoperative cataract surgery regimen to offer corneal analgesia. We now use an NSAID routinely for all cataract surgery patients, preoperatively and postoperatively, mainly to help reduce inflammation and the incidence of cystoid macular edema. A topical fourth-generation fluoroquinolone (Zymar) and a steroid (PredForte) are also part of my medication routine for cataract surgery. We do not patch the eye after LRIs, but we do apply povidone-iodine 5% on the cornea preoperatively and immediately postoperatively.

Measuring Results

A number of methods are available to measure our results with LRIs. Newer computer software includes postoperative astigmatic analysis. Surgically induced refractive change and vector analysis often are used to demonstrate astigmatic change. A simpler way to follow results is to measure the amount of postoperative cylinder at any axis. If a patient has <0.75 D of postoperative astigmatism, he or she is likely to be happy with his or her results.

The Future of Limbal-Relaxing Incisions

Like phacoemulsification, LRI instruments and techniques will continue to evolve. As we follow LRI results with imaging, such as sophisticated corneal topography and wavefront aberrometry, modifications as adjustments in blade depth and optic-zone diameter will help us to improve. Competition with toric IOLs and combinations of bioptics with corneal laser and light-adjustable IOLs may reduce LRI popularity. Femtosecond cataract surgery has tended to validate the benefits of LRIs, and time will tell as to surgeon adoption of this new technology. In the meantime, traditional LRI techniques remain an important ingredient to achieve spectacle reduction with refractive lens–procedures. Regardless, any improvement in methods to reduce unwanted astigmatism will continue to be an important part of successful refractive cataract surgery.

References

1. Osher RH. Consultations in refractive surgery. *J Refract Surg.* 1987;3(6):240.
2. Wallace RB, American Society of Cataract and Refractive Surgery. On-axis cataract incisions: where is the axis? In: Best Papers of Sessions. American Society of Cataract and Refractive Surgery. 1995;67-72.

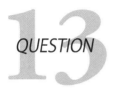

QUESTION

13

MY PATIENTS HAVE IRREGULAR ASTIGMATISM. ARE THEY STILL CANDIDATES FOR A TORIC INTRAOCULAR LENS OR LIMBAL-RELAXING INCISIONS? IF NOT, WHAT ARE MY OPTIONS?

Parag Majmudar, MD and Fred Chu, MD

Several options exist for the management of patients with cataract and irregular astigmatism. However, to provide predictable and successful outcomes, it is important to consider some key principles prior to determining the best course of action.

Determining the Best Course for Optimal Outcomes

STABILITY OF ASTIGMATISM

It is critical to determine the stability of the astigmatic readings. This can be accomplished with serial corneal topography. Documenting stability of a patient's astigmatism increases the likelihood that a refractive procedure will provide long-term benefit. The amount of time over which the astigmatic measurement should be stable prior to refractive surgery is debatable, but certainly the longer the duration of stability, the more predictable the results. A special circumstance is patients with prior penetrating keratoplasty. In this subset, any additional refractive procedure should be deferred until all corneal sutures have been removed and residual astigmatism is shown to be stable over time.

PATIENTS WITH UNSTABLE OR IRREGULAR ASTIGMATISM

Another important variable concerns how orthogonal is the patient's corneal astigmatism. By orthogonal, we mean how close the 2 steep axes are to forming a straight line. In patients who are poor candidates for refractive procedures, rigid gas-permeable (RGP) contact lenses may be a successful option. By virtue of their ability to create a tear meniscus under the lens, RGP contact lenses can compensate for corneal irregularities. Therefore, for patients with unstable or irregular astigmatism, RGP contact lenses may be an excellent choice. Unfortunately, some patients are unable to tolerate contact lenses or lack the dexterity to place them. In these patients, other options must be considered.

REFRACTIVE PROCEDURES THAT CAN IMPROVE IRREGULAR ASTIGMATISM

Several refractive procedures, such as laser in situ keratomileusis (LASIK), astigmatic arcuate keratotomy, and photorefractive keratectomy, can improve irregular astigmatism, even if non-orthogonal. However, one should consider that these procedures can leave the cornea vulnerable to ectasia or other problems if future procedures are required. Furthermore, these techniques are predicated on using topography-guided excimer laser ablation, which is currently not US Food and Drug Administration-approved in the United States. However, a US clinical trial of topography-guided excimer laser ablation (Wavelight T-CAT; Alcon Laboratories) is currently in progress.

If a patient's irregular astigmatism is stable, incisional surgery (eg, arcuate keratotomy) may decrease the magnitude of cylinder. It should be emphasized that RGP contact lenses still may be required for optimal vision postoperatively. However, if the astigmatism is due to an ectatic process, such as keratoconus or post-LASIK ectasia, incisional surgery should be avoided to prevent focal thinning and further ectasia.

DETERMINING WHICH PATIENTS ARE CANDIDATES FOR TORIC INTRAOCULAR LENS

In patients with both cataract and irregular astigmatism, toric intraocular lenses (IOLs) can be an effective strategy.[1,2] However, there are several important considerations when determining which patients with irregular astigmatism will benefit from this option.

First, these IOLs are relatively expensive and provide permanent results. Again, documenting stable corneal topography is critical. In addition, more orthogonal astigmatism allows for more predictable outcomes. In cases where the astigmatism is perfectly orthogonal, the toric IOL should be aligned with that axis. When the axes are near orthogonal, we suggest choosing an axis between the 2 main steep axes. However, as the following example shows, the ideal axis can be difficult to determine, and these cases may benefit from intraoperative aberrometry.

A representative case is provided courtesy of Carlos Buznego, MD, Miami, Florida. A 64-year-old male was seen for cataract consultation. Although his topography was suggestive of forme fruste keratoconus (Figure 13-1), this had been stable for some time, and the decision was made to implant a toric IOL.

Corneal topography revealed +0.88 diopters (D) of astigmatism at the 146-degree meridian. However, automated keratometry (Figure 13-2) revealed +1.12 D of astigmatism at the 165-degree meridian. An Alcon AcrySof IQ toric IOL, model SN60T3, was selected, with planned placement at the 165-degree meridian.

It should be noted that some surgeons might have selected an axis intermediate between the topographic and interferometric axes. During surgery, the IOL was positioned at the 5 degree meridian, 20 degrees counterclockwise of the intended meridian. This is commonly done because the IOL often rotates further during viscoelastic removal, and final adjustments are made after this step. However, in this case, an intraoperative aberrometer (ORA; WaveTec Vision) was used to verify the power and the position of the toric IOL. The aberrometer indicated that the refraction with the lens in the current position at the 5 degree meridian (39 degrees away from the topographic axis) would result in a minimal residual refractive error of +0.38 D cylinder at axis 115 degrees. After this reading was confirmed several times, the IOL was not manipulated further.

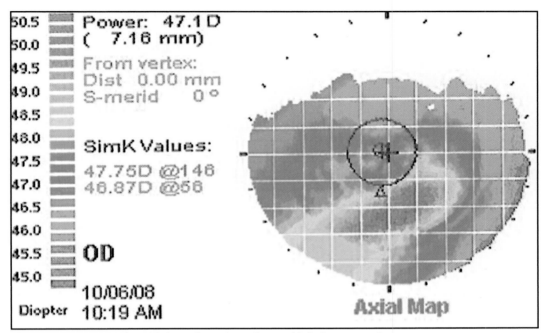

Figure 13-1. Topography with irregular astigmatism and inferior steepening.

OD (right)
K1: 46.75 D at 80°
K2: 48.01 D at 170°
ΔD: +1.26 D at 170°
K1: 46.75 D at 75°
K2: 47.87 D at 165°
ΔD: +1.12 D at 165°
K1: 47.20 D at 78°
K2: 47.94 D at 168°
ΔD: +0.74 D at 168°
n: 1.3375

Figure 13-2. Automated keratometry revealed +1.12 D of astigmatism at the 165-degree meridian.

On postoperative day 5, the toric IOL was well-positioned at the 5 degree meridian. The patient's uncorrected visual acuity was 20/25 in the right eye, and manifest refraction was −0.75 +0.25 x 105, correcting to 20/25[+2]. Most importantly, the patient was "20/happy."

This case shows that current methods of toric IOL axis selection can be unpredictable in cases of irregular astigmatism. This may explain why some patients have significant residual astigmatism after toric IOL placement, and it may make a case for using other technologies for guidance. Care should be taken if selecting a toric IOL for patients who plan to use RGP contact lenses postoperatively. As the tear meniscus created under the contact lens neutralizes corneal astigmatism, use of RGP contact lenses in a patient with a toric lens may result in pseudophakic lenticular astigmatism.

Conclusion

Perhaps the most important consideration in managing patients with irregular astigmatism is to set appropriate expectations. These patients should understand that it may not be possible to achieve spectacles independence and that a goal of improved, but not perfect, best-corrected visual acuity may be more reasonable.

References

1. Navas A, Suárez R. One-year follow-up of toric intraocular lens implantation in forme fruste keratoconus. *J Cataract Refract Surg*. 2009;35(11):2024-2027.
2. Visser N, Gast ST, Bauer NJ, Nuijts RM. Cataract surgery with toric intraocular lens implantation in keratoconus: a case report. *Cornea*. 2011;30(6):720-723.

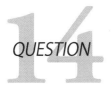
I HAVE A CATARACT PATIENT WITH A TRAUMATIC IRIS DEFECT AND GLARE SYMPTOMS. WHAT SHOULD I DO?

Michael E. Snyder, MD and
Mauricio A. Perez, MD

If the iris defect is clinically significant, cataract surgery alone is not likely to solve the patient's symptoms. Preoperative evaluation provides crucial clues to help determine the defect's clinical relevance.

Preoperative Assessment

When available, a history of iris defect–related photic symptoms present before cataract formation can foreshadow postoperative glare and photophobia. In contradistinction, an absence of previous photic complaints is unreliable in predicting postcataract surgery symptoms because the cataract itself might be acting as a masking factor.

Careful slit-lamp examination aids in assessing other ocular comorbidities commonly seen in iris-defect patients, including zonular weakness, focal vitreous prolapse, and damage to the trabecular meshwork or corneal endothelium.

The nature and extent of the iris defect must be determined, avoiding underestimation based on a misleading initial examination. The iris defect may be anatomic, with absence of, or damage to stromal tissue or function. This may manifest from either muscle or pigment epithelial layer damage. Biomicroscopy of these special patients should be performed both before and after pharmacologic mydriasis because nonmydriatic retroillumination can ascertain whether there might be insufficient pigment to prevent excess light from entering the eye, creating glare, halos, or double images.

Gonioscopy is particularly important for peripheral iris defects or iridodialysis, in which adjacent tissue damage may be masked.

Iris Injuries Less Than 3 Clock-Hours

As a rule of thumb, iris injuries compromising less than 3 clock-hours are candidates for primary iris repair. We prefer 10-0 polypropylene suture to reconstruct remaining native iris tissue by a combination of interrupted sutures using the modified Siepser knot,[1] or peripheral iris reattachment, depending on the anatomy of the original injury.[2]

For single iris sutures, we prefer to use a long, curved needle—we use a 10-0 polypropylene suture on a CTC-6L needle (Ethicon Inc)—entering the eye through a paracentesis. We take the proximal bite of the iris directly, using the needle, and then we use a 25-gauge forceps through a second paracentesis to hold the distal iris in place, taking the second and distal iris bite, then the needle exits the eye through the corneoscleral limbus (Figure 14-1). We encourage the use of the modified Siepser slip knot to secure the sutures on a 2-1-1 fashion. A key surgical pearl is to avoid catching any corneal fibers at the paracentesis when entering the eye with the needle to avoid difficulty with synching the knot down to the iris.

Iris Injuries Greater Than 3 Clock-Hours

Most iris injuries greater than 3 clock-hours require the use of a prosthetic iris device to alleviate a patient's photic symptoms maximally. When possible, we prefer to maintain a small incision, especially in these eyes, which tend to have other comorbidities. Several small-incision iris devices are suitable for placement within an intact capsular bag. The device selection depends on the iris-defect configuration; importance of cosmesis, or lack thereof; availability; and cost.

MORCHER IRIS IMPLANTS

The Morcher Endocapsular Tension Ring 50- and 96-series iris implants (Morcher GmbH) are black PMMA (poly-methyl-methacrylate) devices that can be inserted generally through a 3.2 mm incision (2.0 to 4.5 mm, depending on the model). The implants can achieve great success in limiting the amount of light accessing the posterior segment, although they do not provide a cosmetic improvement (Figure 14-2).

HUMANOPTICS PROSTHESIS

The HumanOptics silicone, flexible iris prosthesis (HumanOptics), customized based on a photo of the fellow eye, provides both excellent functional and cosmetic results (Figure 14-3). Although either passive or scleral-sutured sulcus placement is an alternative, we strongly encourage in-the-bag insertion of the device when the capsule remains intact. This will avoid uveal contact and reduce the risk of device dislocation secondary to late suture hydrolysis.[3]

When using this device, we trephinate the prosthesis to 9.5 mm in diameter for a normal-sized adult eye. For unusually sized anterior segments, we estimate the bag size intraoperatively, using an intraocular ruler (Snyder Ruler; MicroSurgical Technology). We then fold the device into thirds, with the colored portion facing outward and the pseudopupil facing up inside an injection cartridge (Figure 14-4).

Distinguishing the position of the prosthesis relative to the capsule can be challenging due to the lack of contrast of this thin, transparent layer and the opaque device, making capsular staining a crucial step to successful implantation. This can be achieved either by trypan blue (VisionBlue; Dutch Ophthalmic) or indocyanine green (IC-Green; Akorn Inc). We have found that, in cases where we desire decreased capsular elasticity,[4-6] such as the infantile capsule or in a case lacking adequate zonular support, the use of trypan blue is most helpful. We select indocyanine green in

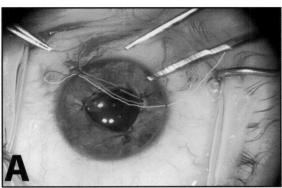

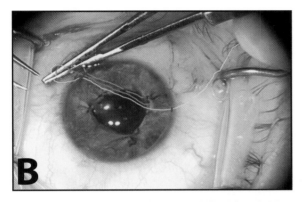

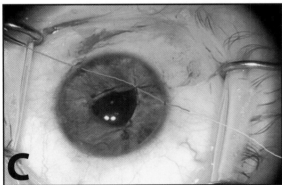

Figure 14-1. (A) The distal portion of the suture (purple and yellow highlighting) is retrieved through the proximal paracentesis (blue) using a Kuglen or similar hook, creating a loop. The strand coming from the iris (purple) should be between the trailing strand (green) and the leading strand (yellow) next to the proximal end of the suture. (B) The forceps is placed from below through the loop, and the trailing strand (green) is placed from above into the forceps tip and grasped. (C) The trailing and leading ends of the suture are pulled, drawing the knot into the anterior chamber and apposing the iris tissue.

cases of native capsular fragility, such as in congenital aniridia, in order to avoid further capsular compromise.[6-8]

Implanting Iris Prosthesis Devices at the Time of Cataract Surgery

Intraocular lens (IOL) power selection in combined phacoemulsification with an in-the-bag iris prosthesis can be challenging due to the posterior shift of the IOL's effective position. We suggest aiming roughly –0.75 diopters more myopic than the intended result to accommodate this shift.

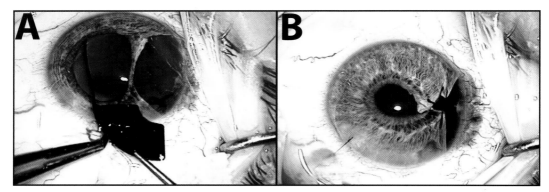

Figure 14-2. (A) In-the-bag insertion and (B) postoperative result of a Morcher Endocapsular tension ring 96 F iris prosthesis.

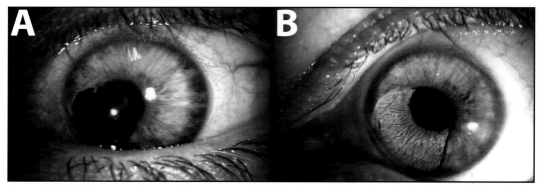

Figure 14-3. (A) Preoperative and (B) postoperative eye using an in-the-bag HumanOptics iris prosthesis.

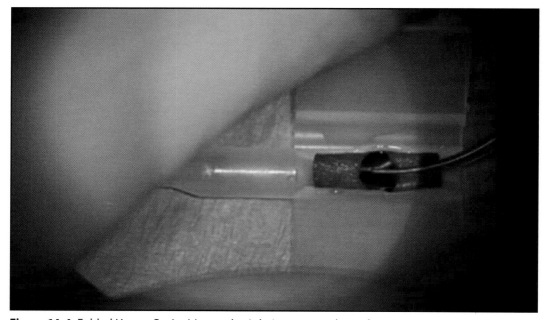

Figure 14-4. Folded HumanOptics iris prosthesis being mounted into the injection cartridge.

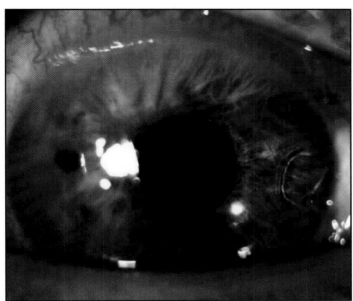

Figure 14-5. In-the-bag Human-Optics iris prosthesis and scleral sutured "Cionni" capsular tension ring.

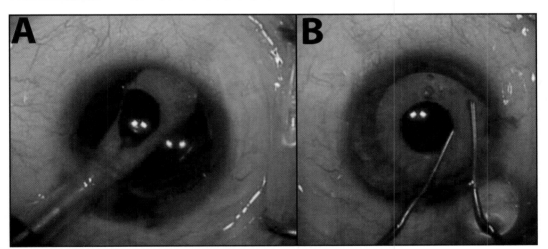

Figure 14-6. (A) Insertion and (B) unfolding of the HumanOptics iris prosthesis.

Phacoemulsification with in-the-bag IOL implantation often must be complemented with zonular support devices as required, whether with standard or scleral-fixated capsular tension rings, capsular tension segments, or both. We recommend securing the bag stability before inserting the iris device (Figure 14-5).

The device is delivered slowly into the bag, anterior to the previously inserted IOL, and 2 Kuglen hooks (Katena Products Inc) are used to unfold it and center it inside the bag (Figure 14-6).

Conclusion

Iris repair at the time of cataract surgery can be a safe and effective treatment for patients with photic symptoms related to an iris defect. The repair technique depends primarily on the amount of iris damage and can range from primary closure for small defects to complete iris prosthetic implants for aniridia. Careful preoperative examination and extensive patient counseling are imperative for successful outcomes.

References

1. Osher RH, Snyder ME, Cionni RJ. Modification of the Siepser slip-knot technique. *J Cataract Refract Surg.* 2005;31(6):1098-1100.
2. Snyder ME, Lindsell LB. Nonappositional repair or iridodialysis. *J Cataract Refract Surg.* 2011;37(4):625-628.
3. Price MO, Price FW Jr, Werner L, Berlie C, Mamalis N. Late dislocation of scleral-sutured posterior chamber intraocular lenses, *J Cataract Refract Surg.* 2005;31(7):1320-1326.
4. Wollensak G, Spörl E, Pham DT. Biomechanical changes in the anterior lens capsule after trypan blue staining. *J Cataract Refract Surg.* 2004;30(7):1526-1530.
5. Dick HB, Aliyeva SE, Hengerer F. Effect of trypan blue on the elasticity of the human anterior lens capsule. *J Cataract Refract Surg.* 2008;34(8):1367-1373.
6. Snyder ME, Osher RH. Evaluation of trypan-blue and indocyanine-green staining of iris prostheses. *J Cataract Refract Surg.* 2011;37(1):206-207.
7. Khng C, Snyder ME. Indocyanine green-emitted fluorescence as an aid to anterior capsule visualization. *J Cataract Refract Surg.* 2005;31(7):1454-1455.
8. Schneider S, Osher RH, Burk SE, Lutz TB, Montione R. Thinning of the anterior capsule associated with congenital aniridia. *J Cataract Refract Surg.* 2003;29(3):523-525.

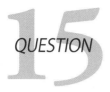

WITH HOW LARGE A ZONULAR DIALYSIS CAN PHACOEMULSIFICATION BE PERFORMED?

Bonnie An Henderson, MD

Surgery in the presence of a zonular dialysis can be a challenging situation for even the most experienced surgeon. The ability to perform small-incision phacoemulsification with a zonular dialysis depends on the density of the lens and the stability and strength of the remaining zonules. If the patient is under the age of 60 and the lens is soft, the nucleus most likely can be removed with slow aspiration (Figure 15-1), even in the presence of a large dialysis, if the remaining intact zonules are strong. Conversely, if the lens is brunescent in the setting of pseudoexfoliation, even a 2 clock-hour dialysis may be too large to complete successful phacoemulsification. The determination of whether to phacoemulsify the lens or to perform a large-incision extraction is based on the combination of both preoperative and intraoperative findings (Table 15-1).

Preoperative Evaluation

The first opportunity to diagnose zonular abnormalities is during the preoperative examination. A careful and thorough history should cover potential risk factors for zonular damage, such as trauma, previous ocular surgery, and systemic conditions such as Marfan syndrome and homocystinuria. A history of prior vitrectomy and chronic silicone-oil tamponade also can be associated with zonular weakness.[1]

At the slit-lamp examination, one should look carefully for pseudoexfoliation. Chamber shallowing, despite a normal axial length, may indicate zonular laxity in such patients.

One method I use to evaluate zonular integrity at the slit lamp is to have the patient look in multiple directions and then straight ahead. If significant zonular weakness exists, one might see phacodonesis during these motility exercises. If phacodonesis is present, it can be assumed that some zonules are weakened. If the contralateral eye is pseudophakic, pseudophacodonesis may

Figure 15-1. Traumatic cataract with zonular dialysis.

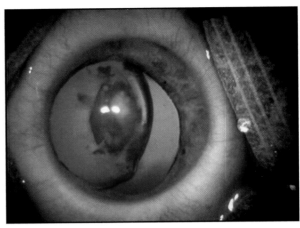

Table 15-1
Stepwise Approach to Evaluation of Zonular Dialysis

1. Careful history (trauma, silicone oil, systemic disease)
2. Preoperative evaluation (pseudoexfoliation, phacodonesis, measurement of anterior chamber depth)
3. Patient consent/counseling
4. Preoperative planning—chondroitin sulfate, capsule staining, capsular hooks, CTRs, scleral tunnel, preoperative NSAID
5. Anesthesia considerations—peribulbar block rather than topical
6. Intraoperative evaluation—movement during capsulorrhexis, phaco
7. Intraoperative procedure—complete hydrodissection, hydrodelineation, supra-capsular approach, use of chopper, placement of hooks, CTRs
8. Plan for conversion to manual extracapsular cataract extraction (ECCE)/intra-capsular cataract extraction/PPV, PPL

Abbreviations: CRTs, capsular tension rings; ECCE, extracapsular cataract extraction; NSAID, nonsteroidal anti-inflammatory drug; PPL, pars plana lensectomy; PPV, pars plana vitrectomy.

indicate the likelihood of zonular weakness in the preoperative eye. Finally, one should dilate the pupil maximally to visualize as much of the peripheral lens as possible.

Preparing the Patient for the Outcome

If zonular weakness is suspected, proper informed consent is crucial in managing the patient's expectations. The patient must be made aware that both the surgery and the postoperative care may be more complicated and prolonged. The patient also should be counseled about the potential need for a vitrectomy, for dislocated lens fragments, and for the greater risk of retinal detachment and cystoid macular edema with vitreous loss. I often will paint the worst-case scenario for patients so they will expect the worst but, hopefully, will be pleasantly surprised.

In cases of zonular dialysis, preoperative planning becomes even more important. In these patients, I will start topical nonsteroidal anti-inflamatory drugs for 3 days preoperatively because of the higher risk for intraoperative complications and postoperative cystoid macular edema. Anticipating a potentially longer operative time, I use peribulbar or retrobulbar anesthesia instead of topical anesthesia in these cases. This also makes it easier to convert to a manual extracapsular cataract extraction (ECCE) if necessary.

In patients where a large zonular dialysis is present, I will perform a scleral tunnel rather than a clear corneal incision to facilitate converting to a large-incision ECCE. The anterior capsule should be stained with trypan blue (Dutch Ophthlamic), especially if capsular hooks are to be used. Of the various viscoelastics, chondroitin sulfate is best suited in cases with a zonular dialysis due to its dispersive, highly retentive properties. The chondroitin sulfate will push back the vitreous face and is not as quickly aspirated. The use of capsular hooks and capsular tension rings will be discussed in Chapter 32.

Intraoperative Assessment

Intraoperative assessment of the degree of zonular dialysis begins when the eye is first manipulated. For example, phacodonesis might be noted during the conjunctival peritomy for preparation of the scleral tunnel incision. The degree of zonular integrity also can be evaluated during the capsulorrhexis. Puncturing the capsule with the cystotome and grasping the flap with the forceps often gives the surgeon an accurate tactile sense of either normal or abnormal countertraction from the zonules. Any improper movement of the lens capsule during hydrodissection or lens sculpting should be noted. Sometimes the zonular laxity is not noted until the lens emulsification has begun. If the lens diaphragm moves posteriorly on attempted lens grooving or chopping, zonular weakness should be suspected.

If a zonular dialysis is present, abundant chondroitin sulfate (dispersive) viscoelastic should be used to prevent anterior prolapse of the vitreous. Capsular hooks and CTRs can be placed before the start of phacoemulsification to stabilize the capsular bag and prevent vitreous prolapse (Figure 15-2).[2-4] The lens must be completely hydrodissected and hydrodelineated to decrease stress on the remaining zonules when the lens is manipulated. If the lens is not fully mobile within the capsular bag, a supracapsular phaco technique should be considered. Avoid a 4-quadrant, divide-and-conquer approach, which necessitates numerous rotations within the capsule. Instead, the use of phaco chopping methods is preferred to minimize stress on the zonules and capsular bag.

SITUATIONS REQUIRING ALTERNATIVE APPROACHES

Zonular dialyses of up to 160 degrees have been reported to have successful outcomes after phacoemulsification with implantation of CTRs.[5] If the dialysis is greater than 5 clock-hours, the lens is brunescent, the pupil dilates poorly, and the integrity of the remaining zonules is compromised, then phacoemulsification of the lens, even with the use of capsular hooks and CTRs, may not be the best approach. In these instances, it may be safer to remove the lens through a large-incision manual extracapsular approach or even with a planned pars plana lensectomy–vitrectomy.

Figure 15-2. Photo of the same lens shown in Figure 15-1 after placement of capsular hooks.

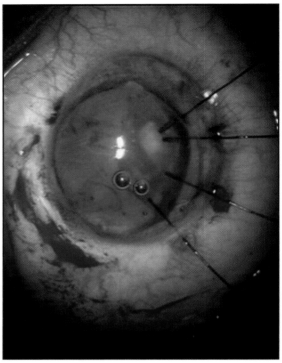

Conclusion

When selecting a surgical approach in the presence of a zonular dialysis, one must consider other ocular variables, such as pupil size, corneal endothelial health, lens density, and the surgeon's familiarity with using capsular hooks and CTRs.

References

1. Menapace R, Findl O, Georgopoulos M, et al. The capsular tension ring: designs, applications, and techniques. *J Cataract Refract Surg.* 2000;26(6):898-912.
2. Hara T, Hara T, Yamada Y. "Equator ring" for maintenance of the completely circular contour of the capsular bag equator after cataract removal. *Ophthalmic Surg.* 1991;22(6):358-359.
3. Legler UFC, Witschel BM. The capsular ring: a new device for complicated cataract surgery. *Ger J Ophthalmol.* 1994;3:265. Abstract F12.
4. Cionni RJ, Osher RH. Management of profound zonular dialysis or weakness with a new endocapsular ring designed for scleral fixation. *J Cataract Refract Surg.* 1998;24(10):1299-1306.
5. Georgopoulos GT, Papaconstantinou D, Georgalas I, et al. Management of large traumatic zonular dialysis with phacoemulsification and IOL implantation using the capsular tension ring. *Acta Ophthalmol Scand.* 2007;85(6):653-657.

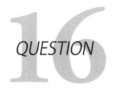
WHEN AND HOW SHOULD I CONSIDER A NONPHACOEMULSIFICATION TECHNIQUE TO REMOVE A CATARACT?

Geoffrey C. Tabin, MA, MD; Dipanjal Dey, MD; and Benjamin Thomas, MD

In the developed world, phacoemulsification currently is the preferred method for cataract extraction; however, it may not always be the best approach for all cataract surgeries. Techniques such as extracapsular cataract extraction and sutureless small-incision cataract surgery (SICS) do not require phacoemulsification to remove cataractous lenses and have specific applications, particularly in the developing world. Lower costs and reduced surgical time make these manual methods ideal in resource-poor settings.[1] Small-incision cataract surgery, in particular, has been adopted widely for its smaller, self-sealing sclero-corneal tunnel (5.5 to 7.0 mm; extracapsular cataract extraction is 10 to 12 mm), reduced complications, and rapid visual recovery.

Small-incision cataract surgery also may be the best approach for selected cataracts in the developed world. Patients with black or brown and morgagnian cataracts, low endothelial cell count, phacolytic glaucoma, shallow anterior chambers, severe pseudoexfoliation, fragile or damaged zonules, and poor visibility through a scarred or vascularized cornea may benefit to a great extent from SICS (Figure 16-1).

Brunescent and Black Cataracts

Small-incision cataract surgery is an excellent procedure for black or very brunescent cataracts. It does not suffer from the limitations and complications associated with phacoemulsification that usually are related to increased surgical time and the ultrasound energy required to break the dense lens typical of advanced cataracts. These extra requirements can lead to endothelial damage and corneal edema.[2] Penetrating and dividing the lens is difficult and may place excessive stress on the bag–zonular complex, which can lead to capsular rupture. Breaking the posterior plate also is very difficult. In contrast, SICS, performed by an experienced surgeon, will take 5 minutes or less for the thickest and blackest of cataracts.[3]

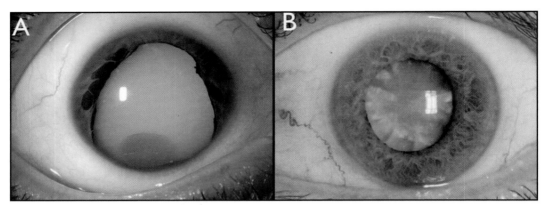

Figures 16-1. Slit-lamp examination of (A) a hypermature, morgagnian cataract with milky cortex surrounding a mobile lens and (B) a brown, advanced cataract.

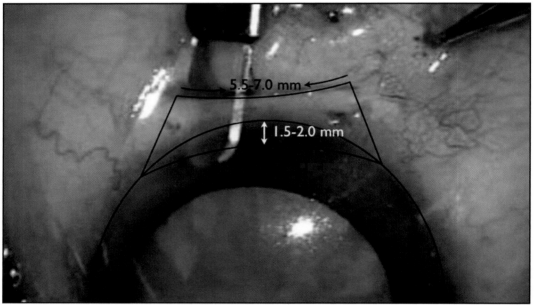

Figure 16-2. Tunnel formation in small-incision cataract surgery. An incision of 5.5 to 7.0 mm in length is made temporally. The wound can extend 1.5 to 2.0 mm into the cornea, providing an inner corneal incision length of approximately 9.0 mm. With maximal extension, a large nucleus can pass through the inner lip of the tunnel.

The incision can be made from either a temporal or a superior approach, depending on the keratometry reading and surgeon preference. The external scleral incision starts 1.5 mm from the limbus and extends 1.5 mm into the clear cornea. The incision should be 5.5 to 7.0 mm in circumferential length, depending on the size of the nucleus, and fan out to 9.0 mm for the internal corneal incision valve, resulting in a conical tunnel with the large cone base facing the anterior chamber and the narrower side toward the incision (Figure 16-2). This architecture allows for smooth delivery of a large nucleus.

A larger nucleus requires a slightly larger incision. After incision and entry, a large continuous curvilinear capsulotomy, with or without relaxing incisions, or a can-opener capsulotomy is

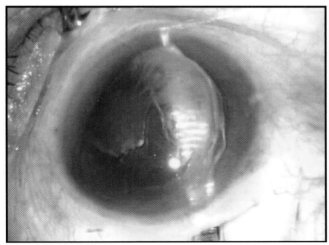

Figure 16-3. Nucleus prolapse using a Simcoe cannula after capsulotomy. The lens is gently lifted into the anterior chamber. Alternative methods include the use of a sinskey hook, hydrodissection, or viscoelastic.

required to provide an exit for the nucleus to be mobilized into the anterior chamber. After capsulorrhexis, the nucleus is gently prolapsed into the anterior chamber by hydrodissection, viscoelastic, with a sinskey hook, or a Simcoe cannula (Figure 16-3). Liberal viscoelastic surrounding the nucleus prevents endothelial injury. This should be performed prior to nucleus expression. The nucleus then is delivered gently out of the eye with viscoelastics or fluid pressure.

Morgagnian Cataracts

Hypermature, morgagnian cataracts often are characterized by weak zonules, tension in the capsular bag, a milky cortex, or a dense mobile nucleus. Capsulorrhexis often is challenging due to a mobile, lax, and fibrotic capsule, as well as cortical pressure. The absence of a protective epinuclear and cortical shell increases the risk of posterior capsular rupture, dropping of nuclear fragments, and zonule dialysis during phacoemulsification.

If continuous curvilinear capsulotomy fails, perform an envelope or V-capsulotomy. After injecting viscoelastic, bring the mobilized nucleus into the anterior chamber bimanually with a spatula or iris repositor from beneath and a sinskey hook from above. Also, the nucleus can be tilted up and the intraocular lens placed into the capsular bag under viscoelastic prior to expression.

Reduced Endothelial Cell Count in the Setting of a Dense Cataract

Patients with endothelial compromise from prior surgery or Fuchs' dystrophy are at risk for pseudophakic bullous keratopathy as a complication of phacoemulsification. The probability of this occurring increases in patients with hard nuclei or shallow anterior chambers.

One way to prevent this adverse result, and endothelial injury in general, is to use abundant viscoelastic to form a soft shell around the lens prior to mobilization. In this approach, a cohesive ophthalmic viscosurgical device is used to form the anterior chamber, and a dispersive ophthalmic viscosurgical device is used to coat the endothelium and surrounding peripheral structures

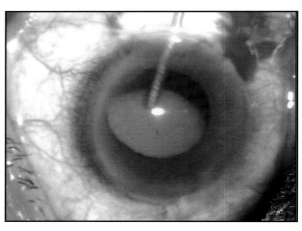

Figure 16-4. A soft-shell technique prevents endothelial injury. A cohesive ophthalmic viscosurgical device is used to form the anterior chamber, and a dispersive viscosurgical device is used to coat the endothelium and surrounding structures to provide protection.

(Figure 16-4). Should the nucleus be large, a larger tunnel can be formed to reduce manipulation during removal, especially with a hard lens.

With the advent of Descemet's stripping automated endothelial keratoplasty, some of these patients may be treated with a combined phacoemulsification/SICS and endothelial corneal transplantation.

Phacolytic Glaucoma

Weakened zonules and poor visualization secondary to anterior chamber lens matter and corneal edema make phacoemulsification a difficult task. Small-incision cataract surgery can be employed with little difficulty after several adjustments. First, one can improve corneal clarity by lowering intraocular pressure with preoperative mannitol or 10 minutes of pressure applied to an anesthetized patient in the peri-retrobulbar block period. Anterior chamber particulate can be cleared using a Simcoe cannula. Capsulotomy techniques are the same as those applied to morgagnian cataracts.

Shallow Anterior Chamber

Maneuvering the phaco tip can be difficult in a shallow anterior chamber. There is a risk of energy-related endothelial damage and Descemet's membrane detachment with phacoemulsification. Small-incision cataract surgery reduces the need for instrumentation and manipulation, thereby improving safety.

Severe Pseudoexfoliation

This condition often is associated with a poorly dilated pupil, posterior synechiae, shallow anterior chambers, hard cataracts, weak zonules, phacodonesis, and subluxated cataracts. It may be best to manage all of these associations with SICS. Here, multiple small sphincterotomies can be used to ease nucleus expression into the anterior chamber.

Zonular Dialysis and Weakness

Nucleus rotation, as well as division and cracking maneuvers, applies significant stress to the zonule fibers and may lead to zonule tears and a dropped nucleus during phacoemulsification. Small-incision cataract surgery may be a safer alternative, especially for the inexperienced surgeon.

Poor Visualization

It may be easier to manage poor visibility with SICS, compared with phacoemulsification, when the view is compromised by corneal opacity or vascularization. The nucleus can be removed easily and safely with SICS, even with a very poor view.

Outcomes

The outcomes of SICS are similar to phacoemulsification, even in uncomplicated cases. Several studies have demonstrated no significant difference in outcomes comparing phacoemulsification with SICS at 6 months in patients with advanced cataracts. Less corneal edema was noted on postoperative day 1 ($P < .004$) and shorter operative times ($P < .0001$) in SICS in a series of very mature cataracts.[3] The complication rates may be higher with phacoemulsification than with manual SICS in the hands of inexperienced surgeons.[4]

Conclusion

SICS may be a good alternative for a wide variety of complicated and advanced cataracts. It is faster, cheaper, less resource-intensive and should be in every surgeon's repertoire.

References

1. Tabin G, Chen M, Espandar L. Cataract surgery for the developing world. *Curr Opin Ophthalmol.* 2008;19(1):55-59.
2. Bourne RR, Minassian DC, Dart JK, et al. Effect of cataract surgery on the corneal endothelium: modern phacoemulsification compared with extracapsular cataract surgery. *Ophthalmology.* 2004;111(4):679-685.
3. Ruit S, Tabin G, Chang D, et al. A prospective randomized clinical trial of phacoemulsification vs manual sutureless small-incision extracapsular cataract surgery in Nepal. *Am J Ophthalmol.* 2007;143(1):32-38.
4. Haripriya A, Chang DF, Reena M, Shekhar M. Complication rates of phacoemulsification and manual small-incision cataract surgery at Aravind Eye Hospital. *J Cataract Refract Surg.* 2012;38(8):1360-1369.

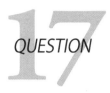

QUESTION

How Do I Incorporate Femtosecond Laser Into My Current Cataract Surgery Techniques?

Richard Tipperman, MD

The femtosecond laser can be utilized to perform several of the most critical steps of cataract surgery. The laser can perform the primary and secondary incisions, arcuate incisions, as well as capsulorrhexis and lens fragmentation.

Advantages of Femtosecond Laser-Assisted Cataract Surgery

Potential advantages of femtosecond laser–assisted cataract surgery include increased precision of arcuate keratotomies, reduced phacoemulsification time, and the ability to produce an essentially perfectly round and centered capsulorrhexis.[1,2] Although the femtosecond laser can be used on most patients undergoing cataract surgery, there are certain patients for whom this technology should offer additional benefits.

Benefits for Patients

Peer-reviewed studies demonstrate an increased ability to target a final postoperative refraction with femtosecond laser–created capsulorrhexis versus a manual capsulorrhexis.[3] This appears to be related to an improved ability to target the effective lens position of the intraocular lens (IOL) implant.

Additional studies have demonstrated that patients with femtosecond laser–created capsulorrhexis have lower degrees of higher-order aberrations, including lens tilt and coma.[4] Higher-order aberrations can degrade the visual quality of patients after cataract surgery, especially those with multifocal IOLs. Other studies[4] have shown that patients with a femtosecond laser–created capsulorrhexis had better Strehl ratios and modulation transfer function when compared with patients who had manually created capsulorrhexis. These findings were all statistically significant.

The Femtosecond Laser in Clinical Practice

Incorporating the femtosecond laser into clinical practice requires the ophthalmologist to make certain of specific assessments during the preoperative clinical evaluation. To be able to use the femtosecond laser, the patient's pupil must dilate widely enough so that the laser can create the capsulorrhexis. In addition, the patient must be able to hold still and cooperate during the procedure.

It is important for the surgeon to measure the dilated pupil size carefully during the preoperative examination. With conventional cataract surgery, if the pupil does not dilate widely enough, the surgeon always has the option to dilate the pupil mechanically. However, mechanical dilation of the pupil is not possible prior to femtosecond laser treatment; therefore, if a patient does not dilate well enough with a maximal pharmacologic regimen, it will not be possible to proceed with femtosecond treatment.

In a similar vein, if a patient has a severe tremor or is unable to cooperate and hold still for conventional cataract surgery, there is always an option of either heavy intravenous sedation or general anesthesia to facilitate the surgical procedure.

It is the preference in our clinic to not sedate patients for femtosecond laser. This is partially related to the logistics of trying to administer anesthesia and monitor a patient within the confines of, and during, a femtosecond laser treatment. It also is related to the significant Bell's phenomenon that patients manifest when sedated. The Bell's phenomenon makes it extremely difficult to achieve adequate exposure and visualization of the corneal surface to allow for "docking" of the femtosecond laser.

The femtosecond laser is incorporated into the actual surgical procedure by completing the laser portion first. The patient is placed in a supine position so that the anterior surface of their cornea is parallel to the floor. For the femtosecond laser to scan the eye with optical coherence tomography (OTC), the laser couples with the ocular surface with a patient interface, also known as a docking device or prism. The patient interface allows the OTC, which is computer-controlled and synchronized with the femtosecond laser, to scan and measure the anterior segment.

By means of a video display, the surgeon can adjust parameters of the surgical treatment so that the femtosecond laser treatment can be customized individually for each patient. These parameters include width, length, and angle of the primary and secondary incisions; arc length and depth of the arcuate incisions; size and centration of the capsulorrhexis; and, last, the pattern that the femtosecond laser uses to fragment the lens. At present, most surgeons are using a cruciate or crossed "X" pattern with or without 1 or 2 concentric rings to fragment the lens. Some surgeons advocate using just concentric rings for softer lenses.

During the capsulorrhexis creation and lens fragmentation, the femtosecond laser creates multiple microbubbles in the anterior chamber. In some surgeries, these bubbles can coalesce and impinge on the iris sphincter and cause pupillary constriction. We have found it helpful in our surgery center to administer a drop of 2.5% or even 10% Neo-synephrine (phenylephrine hydrochloride) following the completion of the laser portion of the procedure, to help maintain excellent pupillary dilation.

Although the actual phacoemulsification portion of the procedure is similar to conventional cataract surgery, there are significant differences. Rather than using a surgical keratome, the incisions can all be opened with a blunt spatula. This helps to preserve the elegant and precise incisional architecture created by the femtosecond laser. In many cases, visual inspection of the anterior capsule reveals that a perfect 360-degree, free-floating rhexis has been achieved. In other cases, despite there being a perfect 360-degree rhexis, the physical separation of the central circular flap is not always obvious and a capsular-type forceps can be used to pull the flap centrally, ensuring completion.

During phacoemulsification, the fragmentation of the lens created by the femtosecond laser markedly facilitates lenticular removal and results in lower phacoemulsification energy use for the cataract surgery.

The postoperative medication regimen and instructions are identical for patients undergoing femtosecond cataract surgery or conventional cataract surgery.

References

1. Nagy ZZ, Kránitz K, Takacs AI, et al. Comparison of intraocular lens decentration parameters after femtosecond and manual capsulotomies. *J Refract Surg.* 2011;27(8):564-569.
2. Kránitz K, Takacs A, Miháltz K, et al. Femtosecond laser capsulotomy and manual continuous curvilinear capsulorrhexis parameters and their effects on intraocular lens centration. *J Refract Surg.* 2011;27(8):558-563.
3. Filkorn T, Kovács I, Knorz MC, et al. Comparison of IOL power calculation and refractive outcome after laser refractive cataract surgery with a femtosecond laser versus conventional phacoemulsification. *J Refract Surg.* 2012;28(8):540-544.
4. Miháltz K, Knorz MC, Alió JL, et al. Internal aberrations and optical quality after femtosecond laser anterior capsulotomy in cataract surgery. *J Refract Surg.* 2011;27(10):711-716.

SECTION II

INTRAOPERATIVE QUESTIONS

How Do I Move From a Larger to a Smaller Phaco Incision?

Paul Ernest, MD

The recent shift toward smaller cataract incisions in phacoemulsification surgery has been prompted by several studies showing less surgically induced astigmatism, quicker stabilization of refraction, and potentially faster healing time, with wounds down to 1.8 mm.[1] As surgeons continue to push the lower limits of coaxial phacoemulsification, they must understand how this will have an impact on the various components of the surgical system. Simply decreasing the size of your keratome without adjusting other aspects of your technique ultimately will lead to failure.

Intraoperative Factors and Challenges

Clinical outcomes of cataract surgery are dependent on many intraoperative factors, including the width and geometry of the surgical wound, the design and diameter of the phacoemulsification apparatus, and the material, shape, and insertion technique of the intraocular lens (IOL). All of these components together constitute the surgical system, and incisions of 1.8 to 2.2 mm require new instrumentation, new phacoemulsification technology, and new IOL designs to maximize the advantages they offer.

The first step to transitioning to a smaller incision is understanding the effects this may have on biometry and lens calculations. Studies have shown not only less surgically induced astigmatism with 2.2-mm wounds over traditional 2.6- to 3.0-mm wounds but also more predictability with lower standard deviations.[1] This makes planning for toric lenses and limbal-relaxing incisions or astigmatic keratotomies easier and ultimately leads to better postoperative refractive results. I have found in my practice that a well-constructed 2.2-mm wound based on the posterior limbus can have surgically induced astigmatism values of 0.25 diopters (D) with a standard deviation of only 0.14 D.

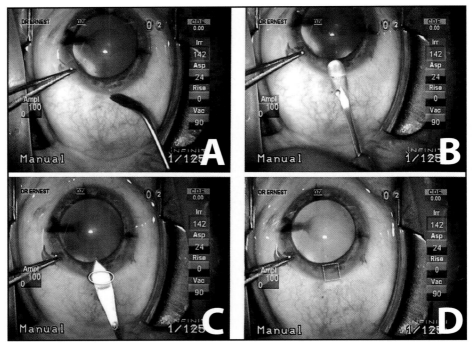

Figure 18-1. Creation of a square posterior limbal incision. (A) Creation of a mechanically sound tri-planar wound begins with a 2.2-mm posterior limbal incision. (B) A crescent blade is used to create a 2.2-mm long pocket from the limbus into the clear cornea. (C) A keratome is used to enter into the anterior chamber. (D) The final result is a square posterior limbal incision with minimal induced astigmatism.

To take advantage of these predictable, low surgically induced astigmatism numbers, one must be meticulous with wound design and execution. A geometrically square wound will be the most mechanically sound, while minimizing the induced astigmatism. Its location is also critical. The closer to the limbus the better.[2] Fibroblasts and elastin fibers found in the limbus aid in quick healing and offer more stretch to the wound, a very important point when dealing with smaller wound sizes.[3]

I prefer to begin my wound with a crescent blade to create a 2.2-mm pocket from the posterior limbus into the clear cornea (Figure 18-1). I then use a keratome to enter the anterior chamber in a controlled maneuver. This ensures a reproducible square wound that seals well.

One of the most challenging parts of cataract surgery with a smaller wound size is the creation of the continuous capsulorrhexis. Intraocular maneuverability is inversely proportional to wound size and necessitates new instruments that take advantage of cross-action mechanics. These instruments allow the surgeon to have greater range with minimal manipulation of the wound. An alternative is to create the capsulorrhexis entirely with the cystitome.

Phacoemulsification techniques remain largely unaffected by smaller wound size; however, the handpiece itself must be sized appropriately to the wound. I prefer a 0.9-mm tapered, 30-degree bevel Kelman tip (Alcon Laboratories), as I find this offers the best compromise of occludability and sculpting power. The use of both traditional ultrasound power and torsional motion is also crucial to minimizing the total energy entering the eye, thus decreasing the chance of wound burns. One also must be mindful of the "occlusion warning" on your phaco machine. Denser lenses have a higher chance of occluding the smaller-bore needle tips and may require removing the probe from the eye and cleaning the tip.

Fluidics will be dictated largely by the decreased phaco-tip diameter. Studies have not found an increased power demand with smaller-caliber instrumentation.[1] Increasing the bottle height will help to offset the potential for decreased flow through the phaco sleeve, as it is pinched by a tighter wound.

Another challenge many surgeons have faced when transitioning to smaller wounds is the increasing difficulty with IOL insertion. Intraocular lens design and insertion technology have advanced rapidly in an attempt to keep up with the ever-shrinking wounds we now make. Despite this effort, many of the commercial injection cartridges are not amenable to direct injection and require tunnel-assisting maneuvers. By placing the cartridge opening over the external wound and maintaining pressure while injecting, the surgeon is able to ensure the wound-tunnel act as an extension of the injector, rather than a barrier. I have found that using a crescent blade to flare the internal wound with lenses over 30.00 D is also helpful, and other surgeons suggest this is helpful for lens powers over 26.00 D.

Wound closure is relatively unchanged and often easier than with traditional larger wounds. Hydration of the wound is rarely necessary to ensure a leak-free close; however, one should be mindful that the internal lip of the wound floor does not roll into the stromal opening.

Conclusion

By decreasing the size of cataract incisions, many surgeons have taken advantage of increasingly predictable postoperative refractions, while maintaining surgical efficiency. A key to making the transition is understanding that a change in wound size early in the surgery can influence your techniques throughout the course of the operation. Ignoring this can lead to intraoperative complications and surgeon frustration.

References

1. Luo L, Lin H, He M, et al. Clinical evaluation of three incision size-dependent phacoemulsification systems. *Am J Ophthalmol.* 2012;153(5):831-839.e2
2. Ernest PH, Neuhann T. Posterior limbal incision. *J Cataract Refract Surg.* 1996;22(1):78-84.
3. Ernest P, Tipperman R, Eagle R, et al. Is there a difference in incision healing based on location? *J Cataract Refract Surg.* 1998;24(4):482-486.

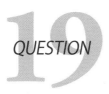

UNDER TOPICAL ANESTHESIA, THE PATIENT IS UNCOOPERATIVE AND COMPLAINING OF PAIN. WHAT SHOULD I DO?

Scott Greenbaum, MD

Cataract surgery can create pain in one or all of 3 ways: (1) manipulation of the ocular surface with sharp instruments or cautery, (2) manipulation or stretching of the iris or ciliary body directly or through overfilling the eye with irrigation fluid or viscoelastic material, and (3) intense halogen microscope illumination. Topical anesthesia effectively blocks the surface of the globe, which is innervated by the frontal branch of the ophthalmic division of the trigeminal nerve, but ignores the other 2 forms of pain signals carried by the nasociliary branch. Although the most common approach to complaint is increased intravenous sedation, it is preferable to ask the patient what is bothering them before signaling to the certified registered nurse anesthetist that you would prefer the patient to receive more sedation, which renders the patient less able to answer.

Approaches to Managing the Patient's Pain

Lowering the infusion bottle or turning down the microscope light might improve the patient's experience enough to continue without intervention. Both, however, can have an impact on the surgeon's performance and the safety of the operation. It is also important to ask the patient directly, or through an interpreter, if their distress is due to a need to urinate. If so, a hand-held urinal should be provided by the circulating nurse or they should be instructed to void on the table.

If none of these approaches apply, the safety of injecting 0.50 cc of unpreserved 1% lidocaine (Abbott Laboratories) into the anterior chamber is well documented.[1] Of course, this is not the answer if intraocular lidocaine or lidocaine gel has already been administered, as gel absorbance, according to work by Koch,[2] provides an anesthetic effect similar to intracameral lidocaine administration.

With these considerations taken, it may still be necessary to restore patient cooperation and immediately cease his or her complaints. You must deliver comfort, no matter the cause of the

Figure 19-1. Greenbaum cannula with opening on its lower surface.

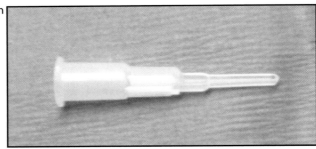

discomfort. Taking the time to have the possibly sedated patient describe the quality and location of the pain experienced is potentially hazardous in the middle of a phacoemulsification. A para-bulbar, or anterior sub-Tenon's block, delivered with a blunt cannula in a way that allows forward progress of the anesthetic mixture without retrograde leakage, is the most efficient solution for this problem.

Anterior sub-Tenon's anesthesia is as old as Turnbull's first description in 1884.[3] He made a cut through conjunctiva and Tenon's capsule, dropped cocaine into it, and found that his patients were more comfortable than those enucleated with Knapp's retrobulbar technique.[4] I have tried Turnbull's technique using a Westcott scissors (Katena Products Inc) and an irrigating cannula. I have tried every metal cannula invented for sub-Tenon's anesthesia. They all leak to some degree, limiting their effect and reducing or eliminating the degree of resulting amaurosis.

Administered without significant leakage, 1.25 mL of a 50/50 mixture of 4% lidocaine (2% may be used if 4% is unavailable, with similar results) and 0.75% bupivacaine (Abbott Laboratories), mixed with Hylenex (recombinant hyaluronidase) (Halozyme Inc) 150 USP [United States Pharmacopeia] units, if available, will produce near-immediate (within 30 seconds) anesthesia and amaurosis soon after (within 1 minute). If it is not available, I do not use animal-derived hyal-uronidase, due to risk of allergic reaction filling the orbit in the presence of an open globe. With one injection, both main ocular sources of patient distress are blocked.

The cannula I have designed for this purpose, the Greenbaum anesthesia cannula, is manu-factured by Alcon Laboratories. It features an expanded hub that serves as a stopcock that blocks the opening in Tenon's capsules created by the 1-snip incision with a Bonn forceps (Katena) and Vannas scissors (Katena Products Inc) for its introduction. It is best to pick a relatively avascular area 3 to 5 mm posterior to the limbus and to reduce vascularity further with gentle cautery. The fused conjunctiva and Tenon's capsule should bunch up toward the cautery tip, which should never be pressed down on the ocular surface for this purpose. I usually choose the inferonasal quadrant, but any of the 4 quadrants can be used. You should not introduce any cannula directly over a rectus muscle. Figure 19-1 illustrates the cannula with its opening on its lower surface. With a fast push, an anesthetic fluid, through hydraulic dissection, will make its way from the blocked opening in Tenon's toward the only other opening, in posterior Tenon's capsule, through which passes the optic nerve. I have demonstrated on a magnetic resonance imaging study that the optic nerve sheath is illuminated on a T2 image by anesthetic fluid delivered in this manner.[5] This technique is best illustrated online at http:// www.youtube.com/watch?v=-pEZ64CGfzE.

If the Greenbaum cannula is unavailable, my next choice is the BD Visitec Sub-Tenon's anes-thesia cannula (#585176; Becton and Dickinson). At 25 mm, it is 15 mm longer than necessary (Figure 19-2); it is the next best cannula available for preventing backflow. However, its length endangers the optic nerve, posterior staphylomas, and other areas of scleral weakness, such as around scleral buckles, if the cannula is inserted to the hub.

The technique that advances a cannula past the equator is called posterior sub-Tenon's anesthe-sia, which shares all of the risks of retrobulbar and parabulbar, including ophthalmic perforation,

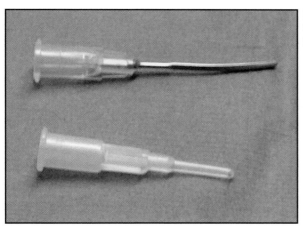

Figure 19-2. Greenbaum cannula and the BD Visitec Sub-Tenon's anesthesia cannula. Note increased length of latter cannula.

optic nerve trauma, and ocular muscle trauma, albeit less commonly. If the longer cannula is to be used, it should be introduced only halfway into the smallest nick of an incision that can be made with a Vannas scissors through a cauterized area identical to the one used in the linked video. It is important to see bare sclera in the floor of the incision site, to attach the cannula to a 3-cc syringe, and to push 1.25 mL of the same anesthetic solution through the incision. With either cannula, the seal can be made tighter and more effective by pulling any loose conjunctiva or Tenon's capsule over the cannula hub or by placing the body of the syringe flush to the globe.

After the opening is made, it can be used at the end of the procedure case to deliver sub-Tenon's antibiotics or steroid. It does not have to be closed, as it will self-seal within days. This site has never been a source of postoperative complaint in my 20 years of experience with the technique.

Conclusion

Have a couple of cannulas and cautery on hand whenever performing topical anesthesia, because a parabulbar or sub-Tenon's block is a safe and effective way to provide fast and effective relief from pain and photophobia experienced during topical anesthesia.

References

1. Martin RG, Miller JD, Cox CC 3rd, Ferrel SC, Raanan MG. Safety and efficacy of intracameral injections of unpreserved lidocaine to reduce intraocular sensation. *J Cataract Refract Surg.* 1998;24(7):961-963.
2. Koch PS. Efficacy of lidocaine 2% jelly as a topical agent in cataract surgery .*J Cataract Refract Surg.* 1999;25(5):632-634.
3. Turnbull CS. Editorial. *Med Surg Rep.* 1884;29:628.
4. Knapp H. On cocaine and its use in ophthalmic surgery. *Arch Ophthalmol.* 1884;13:402.
5. Greenbaum S. Anesthesia for cataract surgery. In: Greenbaum S, ed. *Ocular Anesthesia.* Philadelphia, PA: WB Saunders; 1997:31.

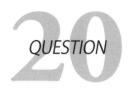
WHAT IS THE BEST WAY TO MANAGE INTRAOPERATIVE FLOPPY IRIS SYNDROME?

David F. Chang, MD

Intraoperative floppy iris syndrome (IFIS), in association with current or prior tamsulosin (Flomax) use, was first described in 2005.[1] Besides a tendency for poor preoperative pupil dilation, severe IFIS exhibits a triad of intraoperative signs: iris billowing and floppiness, iris prolapse to the main- and side-port incisions, and progressive intraoperative miosis (Figure 20-1).

A wide range of clinical severity can be seen in clinical practice. If surgeons do not recognize or anticipate IFIS, the rate of reported intraoperative complications increases.[2-6] Complications of iris prolapse or aspiration include iridodialysis, iris sphincter damage, hyphema, and significant iris stromal or transillumination defects.

In 2009, a retrospective Canadian study of nearly 100,000 cataract surgeries on males documented a doubling of the rate of serious postoperative complications, including retinal detachment, retained nuclear fragments, and severe inflammation in tamsulosin patients.[6] In a 2008 American Society of Cataract Refractive Surgery (ASCRS) membership survey, despite widespread recognition of IFIS at the time, 95% of the respondents still reported that tamsulosin increased the difficulty of cataract surgery, and 77% also believed that it increased the risk of complications.[3] Specifically, during the prior 2 years, IFIS had increased the rate of posterior capsular rupture for 52% of respondents and the rate of significant iris trauma for 23% of the respondents.

Pharmacology and Mechanism of Intraoperative Floppy Iris Syndrome

All alpha-1 antagonists may inhibit pupil dilation and cause IFIS.[4] A number of retrospective and prospective studies, however, have shown that the frequency and severity of IFIS is much higher with tamsulosin, as compared with nonselective alpha-1 antagonists.[1-8] For example, the

Figure 20-1. Severe IFIS: iris billowing, prolapse to phaco and side-port incision, and pupil constriction in a patient taking tamsulosin.

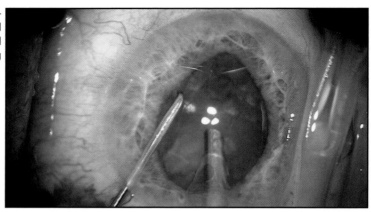

large retrospective Canadian study previously discussed reported that tamsulosin significantly increased the rate of postoperative complications but that nonselective alpha antagonists did not.[6]

A second Canadian retrospective study found that 86% of patients taking tamsulosin developed IFIS, compared with only 15% of patients taking alfuzosin (Uroxatral).[5] A prospective masked trial from Italy[7] comparing phaco in patients taking tamsulosin versus nonselective alpha blockers and a large 2011 meta-analysis[8] of the literature reached this same conclusion: IFIS is more common and severe with tamsulosin. Intraoperative floppy iris syndrome also may occur in patients without any history of alpha antagonist use, and it has been correlated with systemic hypertension in the absence of alpha blockers.

The mechanism of IFIS is not fully understood. In the publication, Chang and Campbell[1] hypothesized that IFIS was a manifestation of decreased iris dilator muscle tone and loss of intraoperative structural rigidity. Two separate slit-lamp optical coherence tomography studies have reported significant thinning of the mid-iris stromal thickness in tamsulosin patients when compared with control eyes.[9] Another widespread finding is that IFIS can occur more than 1 year after tamsulosin has been discontinued.[1-4] A large histopathologic study of autopsy eyes from patients taking tamsulosin (26 eyes) also showed atrophy of the iris dilator muscle, which was consistent with a permanent drug effect on iris morphology.[10]

In 2012, Goseki et al[11] published their in vitro and histologic rabbit studies showing longer-term smooth-muscle degeneration relating to tamsulosin accumulation in adjacent iris-pigment epithelial cells. These permanent structural changes would explain the occurrence of IFIS long after tamsulosin cessation. A stronger binding affinity to iris-pigment granules and alpha-1A receptors might explain the greater propensity for tamsulosin to cause IFIS compared with nonselective alpha antagonists. Finally, the strong affinity for some systemic medications, such as psychotropic drugs, to bind to iris-pigment granules might explain the occasional occurrence of IFIS in patients who have never taken alpha antagonists.

Clinical and Surgical Management of Intraoperative Floppy Iris Syndrome

PREOPERATIVE MANAGEMENT

The possibility of IFIS increases the importance of taking the patient's medication history prior to cataract surgery. A history of systemic alpha antagonists may not be elicited without direct questioning about current or prior use of prostate medication.[3]

Stopping tamsulosin preoperatively is of unpredictable and questionable value. With so many reported cases of IFIS occurring up to several years after the drug had been stopped, it is clear that ophthalmologists cannot rely solely on drug cessation to prevent this condition.

In a multicenter prospective trial, tamsulosin was discontinued prior to surgery in 19% of patients but did not result in any significant reduction in IFIS severity in this subgroup of eyes.[2] In the 2008 ASCRS IFIS survey,[3] 64% of respondents said they never stop tamsulosin prior to surgery, compared with 11% who routinely do.

Preoperative atropine drops (eg, 1%, 3 times per day for 1 to 2 days preoperatively) can enhance cycloplegia as a means of preventing intraoperative miosis.[4] However, the multicenter prospective tamsulosin study[2] demonstrated that atropine, as a single strategy, is often ineffective for more severe cases of IFIS. In the ASCRS IFIS survey,[3] 57% of respondents said that they never use topical atropine prior to surgery, compared with 19% who routinely do.

SURGICAL MANAGEMENT

The inter-individual variability in the severity of IFIS makes it difficult to determine whether one surgical strategy is superior to another.[4] The severity of IFIS is likely to be greater in patients taking tamsulosin.[1-8] Poor preoperative pupil dilation and billowing of the iris immediately following instillation of intracameral lidocaine are also predictive of greater IFIS severity.[2,4,8] In contrast, if the pupil dilates well preoperatively, mild to moderate IFIS is more likely; however, the surgeon should still be prepared for iris prolapse and miosis. Patients taking nonselective alpha-1 antagonists or who already have discontinued these medications for several months are most likely to display mild to moderate IFIS.

Ideally, surgeons should be facile with several different approaches that may be used alone or in combination to manage the iris in IFIS. In general, one should make a constructed, shelved, clear, corneal incision; perform hydrodissection very gently; and consider reducing the irrigation and aspiration flow parameters, if possible. Partial-thickness sphincterotomies and mechanical pupil stretching are ineffective for IFIS and may worsen the iris prolapse and miosis.[1,4]

Intracameral injection of alpha agonists, such as phenylephrine or epinephrine, is a safe and inexpensive strategy for IFIS.[12-15] By presumably saturating the alpha-1A receptors, these agonists can further dilate the pupil (Figure 20-2). It may take a minute before the pupil slowly dilates further; however, if it does not, the alpha agonist often will increase iris dilator muscle tone, reducing billowing and the tendency for prolapse or sudden miosis. Because of the variable severity of IFIS, intracameral alpha agonists work well in some eyes but may have no detectable effect in others.[4]

In the United States, preservative-free 1:1000 epinephrine is packaged in single-use, 1-mL vials (1 mg/mL) and comes in two forms—with and without 0.1% bisulfite as a stabilizing agent. Bisulfite improves the stability of the solution by delaying oxidation of the active substance, but it is toxic to the corneal endothelium due to its high buffer capacity. In addition, epinephrine taken directly from the vial has a low pH of approximately 3.0. Therefore, direct intracameral injection of undiluted 1:1000 epinephrine should be avoided. Instead, a 1:4 epinephrine dilution can be constituted easily by adding 0.2 mL of commercially available 1:1000 epinephrine to 0.8 mL of

Figure 20-2. Tamsulosin patient with pupil diameter (A) before and (B) after intracameral injection of 1:4000 unpreserved epinephrine mixture.

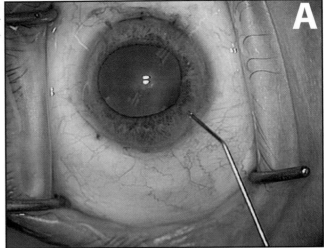

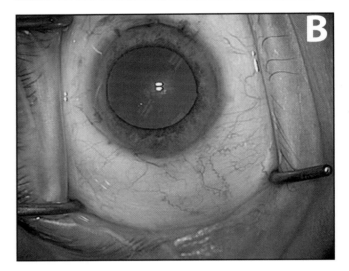

plain balanced salt solution (BSS) or BSS Plus in a 3-mL disposable syringe. This dilution raises the pH to a physiologic level and appears to dilute the bisulfite stabilizing agent sufficiently.[12,14]

Although bisulfite-free 1:1000 epinephrine is theoretically preferred for intracameral injection, there has been a nationwide shortage in the United States at the time of this writing. The 1:4 dilution of bisulfite-containing epinephrine has been used safely by the author and was endorsed in a 2013 ASCRS clinical alert for use when bisulfite-free epinephrine is unavailable. Adding bisulfite-containing epinephrine to a 500-mL BSS irrigation bottle, off label, will not cause corneal endothelial toxicity because of the significant dilution. However, shortages even of bisulfite-containing 1:1000 epinephrine are currently being reported in the United States. The author has noted an increased incidence of IFIS, despite the absence of systemic alpha antagonists whenever epinephrine is omitted from the BSS irrigation bottle.

Several publications report the safety and efficacy of unpreserved 1.5% intracameral phenylephrine for both IFIS prevention and routine surgical mydriasis.[13-15] Preservative-free phenylephrine 2.5% (Minims) is only commercially available outside of the United States. Because these preparations still contain bisulfite, a 1:4 dilution with BSS, BSS Plus, or preservative-free lidocaine also

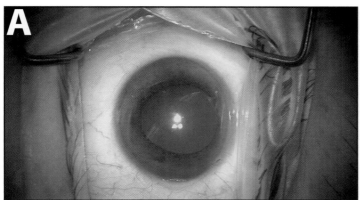

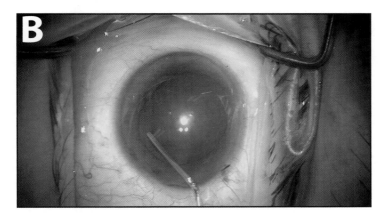

Figure 20-3. (A) Pupil in patient taking tamsulosin is not dilated well even after intracameral epinephrine administration. (B) Healon5 widens the pupil diameter prior to the capsulorrhexis step.

is recommended. Lacking a commercial source in the United States, many surgeons, including the author, obtain bisulfite-free intracameral phenylephrine 1.5% prepared by compounding pharmacies. To avoid potential toxicity from preservative-containing phenylephrine, ophthalmologists should specify that only the unpreserved (raw) drug should be used as a compounding source. Prudent precautions for any drug compounded for intracameral injection include appropriate testing for pH, osmolality, and sterility. Ophthalmologists should check to see if the compounding pharmacy is accredited by the Pharmacy Compounding Accreditation Board.

Healon5 (Abbott Medical Optics Inc) is a maximally cohesive ophthalmic viscosurgical device that is particularly well-suited for viscomydriasis and for blocking iris prolapse in IFIS[2,4] (Figure 20-3A). If mydriasis is still suboptimal after injecting epinephrine, Healon5 then can be used to expand the pupil further mechanically (Figure 20-3B). Viscomydriasis facilitates the capsulorrhexis and combines with the epinephrine-induced iris rigidity to block iris prolapse. However, to avoid immediately aspirating Healon5, one must employ low flow and vacuum parameters (eg, <175 to 200 mm Hg; <26 mL/min).[2,4] This strategy is therefore less suitable if high vacuum settings are desired for denser nuclei. At higher aspiration flow rates, others have suggested that more dispersive ophthalmic viscosurgical devices, such as DisCoVisc (Alcon Laboratories) or VISCOAT (Alcon Laboratories), may persist for longer periods within the eye.

Mechanical pupil expansion with iris retractors or devices, such as the Malyugin Ring (MicroSurgical Technology) discussed in Chapter 21, assures a reliably wide pupil diameter that cannot constrict abruptly during surgery (Figure 20-4).[1-4,16,17] If one uses iris hooks, reusable 4-0 polypropylene retractors (Katena Products Inc and FCI Ophthalmics Inc, respectively) are more rigid and easier to manipulate when compared with 6-0 nylon retractors. Furthermore,

Figure 20-4. Malyugin Ring in eye with IFIS. The floppy iris is still able to prolapse to the incision, but the pupil cannot constrict.

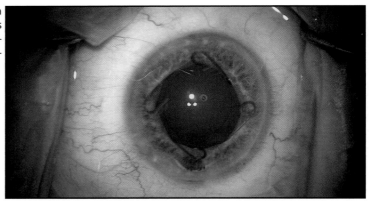

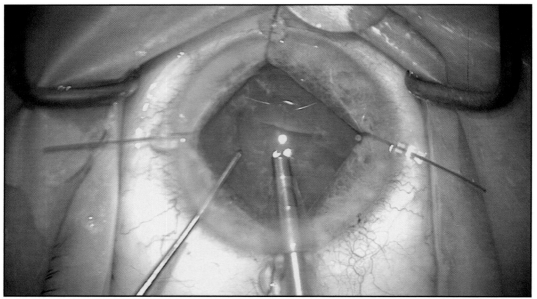

Figure 20-5. 4–0 polypropylene iris retractors are stiffer and easier to manipulate than 6-0 nylon retractors. A separate limbal stab incision is made just behind the temporal clear corneal incision and angled toward the pupil margin. Unlike with pseudoexfoliation, posterior synechiae, or chronically miotic pupils, the IFIS pupil stretches without tearing and can be dilated maximally. When placed in a diamond configuration, the subincisional retractor pulls the iris down and away from the phaco tip. The phaco tip slides above the subincisional retractor lying within a separate tunnel, while the nasal retractor maximizes surgical exposure for the chopper.

4-0 polypropylene hooks can be autoclaved repeatedly in the supplied storage case, which makes them more cost effective than disposable hooks or pupil expansion rings. Placing the hooks in a diamond configuration has several advantages[17] (Figure 20-5). The subincisional hook retracts the iris downward and out of the path of the phaco tip. This provides excellent access to subincisional cortex and avoids tenting the iris in front of the phaco tip, such as occurs when the retractors are placed in a square configuration. This configuration also maximizes temporal exposure directly in front of the phaco tip, as well as nasal exposure for placement of the chopper tip.

Mechanical devices also permit surgeons to use their preferred ophthalmic viscosurgical device, phaco technique, and fluidic parameters. It is easier and safer to insert these devices prior to creation of the capsulorrhexis. If the pupil dilates poorly preoperatively (eg, 3- to 5-mm diameter) or billows during injection of intracameral lidocaine, one should consider proceeding directly to mechanical devices due to of the likelihood of severe IFIS. If the pupil dilates well preoperatively but begins to constrict or prolapse after hydrodissection or during phaco, combining intracameral epinephrine and Healon5 can be an excellent rescue technique that may avoid the need to insert mechanical devices. If iris retractors are used, one should retract the pupil margin with a second instrument to avoid hooking the capsulorrhexis margin with the retractors.

Conclusion

Eliciting a history of current or prior alpha-1 antagonist use should alert surgeons to anticipate IFIS and to employ these strategies either alone or in combination. Because of the variability in IFIS severity, many surgeons use a staged management approach.[4] Pharmacologic measures alone may be sufficient for mild to moderate IFIS cases. Even if they fail to enlarge the pupil, intracameral alpha agonists can reduce or prevent iris billowing and prolapse by increasing iris-dilator muscle tone. If the pupil diameter is still inadequate, viscomydriasis with Healon5 can further expand it for the capsulorrhexis step. Finally, mechanical expansion devices assure the best surgical exposure for severe IFIS and should be considered when other risk factors, such as weak zonules or a brunescent nucleus, are present.

References

1. Chang DF, Campbell JR. Intraoperative floppy iris syndrome associated with tamsulosin (Flomax). *J Cataract Refract Surg.* 2005;31(4):664-673.
2. Chang DF, Osher RH, Wang L, Koch DD. Prospective multicenter evaluation of cataract surgery in patients taking tamsulosin (Flomax). *Ophthalmology.* 2007;114(5):957-964.
3. Chang DF, Braga-Mele R, Mamalis N, et al; ASCRS Cataract Clinical Committee. Clinical experience with intraoperative floppy-iris syndrome. Results of the 2008 ASCRS member survey. *J Cataract Refract Surg.* 2008;34(7):1201-1209.
4. Chang DF, Braga-Mele R, Mamalis N, et al; clinical review of ASCRS Cataract Clinical Committee. ASCRS White Paper: intraoperative floppy iris syndrome. *J Cataract Refract Surg.* 2008;34(12):2153-2162.
5. Blouin MC, Blouin J, Perreault S, Lapointe A, Dragomir A. Intraoperative floppy iris syndrome associated with alpha-1 adrenoreceptors: comparison of tamsulosin and alfuzosin. *J Cataract Refract Surg.* 2007;33(7):1227-1234.
6. Bell CM, Hatch WV, Fischer HD, et al. Association between tamsulosin and serious ophthalmic adverse events in older men following cataract surgery. *JAMA* 2009;301(19):1991-1996.
7. Chatziralli IP, Sergentanis TN. Risk factors for intraoperative floppy iris syndrome: a meta-analysis. *Ophthalmology.* 2011;118(4):730-735.
8. Casuccio A, Cillino G, Pavone C, Spitale E, Cillino S. Pharmacologic pupil dilation as a predictive test for the risk of intraoperative floppy-iris syndrome. *J Cataract Refract Surg.* 2011;37(8):1447-1454.
9. Prata TS, Palmiero PM, Angelilli A, et al. Iris morphologic changes related to alpha(1)-adrenergic receptor antagonists implications for intraoperative floppy iris syndrome. *Ophthalmology.* 2009;116(5):877-881.
10. Santaella RM, Destafeno JJ, Stinnett SS, et al. The effect of alpha1-adrenergic receptor antagonist tamsulosin (Flomax) on iris dilator smooth muscle anatomy. *Ophthalmology.* 2010;117(9):1743-1749.
11. Goseki T, Ishikawa H, Ogasawara S, et al. Effects of tamsulosin and silodisin on isolated albino and pigmented rabbit iris dilators: possible mechanism of intraoperative floppy-iris syndrome. *J Cataract Refract Surg.* 2012;38(9):1643-1649.

12. Shugar JK. Use of epinephrine for IFIS prophylaxis [letter]. *J Cataract Refract Surg.* 2006;32(7):1074-1075.

13. Gurbaxani A, Packard R. Intracameral phenylephrine to prevent floppy iris syndrome during cataract surgery in patients on tamsulosin. *Eye (Lond).* 2007;21(3):331-332.

14. Myers WG, Edelhauser HF. Shortage of bisulfite-free preservative-free epinephrine for intracameral use. *J Cataract Refract Surg.* 2011;37(3):611.

15. Lorente R, de Rojs V, Vázquez de Parga P, et al. Intracameral phenylephrine 1.5% for prophylaxis against intraoperative floppy iris syndrome: prospective, randomized fellow eye study. *Ophthalmology.* 2012;119(10):2053-2058.

16. Chang DF. Use of Malyugin pupil expansion device for intraoperative floppy iris syndrome: results in 30 consecutive cases. *J Cataract Refract Surg.* 2008;34(5):835-841.

17. Oetting TA, Omphroy LC. Modified technique using flexible iris retractors in clear corneal cataract surgery. *J Cataract Refract Surg.* 2002;28(4):596-598.

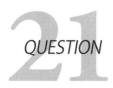

MY PATIENT HAS A SMALL PUPIL. WHAT ARE MY OPTIONS FOR EXPANSION?

Boris Malyugin, MD, PhD

In many cases, poor pupillary dilation during cataract surgery can be anticipated preoperatively. It is seen often in patients with a history of glaucoma, pseudoexfoliation syndrome, uveitis, trauma, or previous intraocular surgery. In addition, a patient who is taking oral alpha-1A antagonists can be expected to exhibit intraoperative floppy iris syndrome (IFIS), which is thought to be the result of iris-sphincter, smooth-muscle atrophy.

Inadequate pupil dilation impairs visualization of the lens and the capsule at all stages of phacoemulsification. In addition, in IFIS patients, there is iris floppiness, or loss of tone, leading to a tendency of the iris to prolapse through the main incision or paracentesis with progressive intraoperative pupil constriction. These factors make surgery challenging and increase the risk for adverse effects and complications.

Dilating the Pupil

In small-pupil patients, I advise using the following sequential stepwise approach: injection of mydriatic into the anterior chamber, utilization of highly viscous ophthalmic viscosurgical device (OVD), lens–iris adhesions separation or peripupillary membranectomy followed by iris stretching. If all of these maneuvers are not effective enough to provide an adequate pupil aperture, then one must consider using a mechanical pupil expander.

Pharmacological therapy with topical nonsteroidal eye drops or strong mydriatics, such as phenylephrine 10%, is effective when administered preoperatively. Nevertheless, it cannot provide an adequate pupil aperture in all patients, especially in the presence of posterior synechiae or a fibrotic pupillary membrane.

Figure 21-1. Mechanical stretching of the pupil with two instruments.

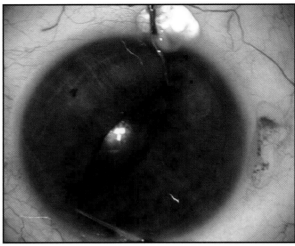

DILATING THE PUPIL WITH PHARMACOLOGICAL AGENTS

Intracameral injection of alpha agonists, such as epinephrine or phenylephrine, at the very beginning of the surgical procedure is extremely effective and a safe addition to topical medications. It is especially beneficial in cases of IFIS. A commonly used concentration of epinephrine is 1:1000 mixed 1:3 with balanced salt solution.

DILATING THE PUPIL MECHANICALLY

If pharmacological agents fail, the surgeon can use an array of techniques and maneuvers to dilate the pupil mechanically. There are 4 main mechanical pupil dilatation methods: synechiolysis, iris stretching, cutting, and retraction.

Adhesions between the iris, lens capsule and/or cornea are usually the result of inflammation or trauma. To release the iris and improve pupil dilation, the adhesions should be lysed. A cyclodialysis spatula or OVD cannula are the most useful instruments to separate adhesions between the lens and the iris. Mechanical separation can be augmented with a small bolus of OVD injection under the iris. In the presence of strong fibrotic tissue, I prefer to use 23- or 25-gauge scissors introduced through the main incision or one of the paracenteses.

The OVD is another tool to be considered in small pupil cases. Viscomydriasis has 2 main components: deepening of the anterior chamber, resulting in pupil dilation, and stabilization of the iris tissue, by placing it in a viscous fluid environment. To achieve these two goals a high-viscosity OVD, such as Healon5 (Abbott Medical Optics Inc) is used. Unfortunately, due to the rheological properties of this device, its sole use requires repeated injections during the ultrasonic lens fragmentation. Alternatively, the surgeon can replace it with a dispersive OVD during phacoemulsification or use the modified iris stabilization method based on creating a donut-shaped layer of Healon5 over the iris, combined with filling of the central portion of the anterior chamber with dispersive OVD (Viscoat; Alcon Laboratories). The latter prevents Healon5 from aspiration.

Mechanical stretching with two instruments (microhooks and microforks) or a special iris dilatator is a relatively simple and effective maneuver (Figure 21-1). This stretching is extremely helpful in small pupils associated with the increased rigidity of a tight iris sphincter. This maneuver creates micro-iris tears that enlarge the pupillary aperture but may also cause bleeding intra- or postoperatively, resulting in an enlarged atonic pupil. It is to be emphasized that stretching of the

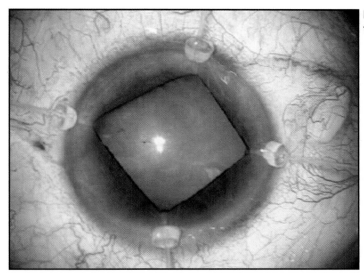

Figure 21-2. Four iris hooks placed to enlarge the pupil.

pupil is ineffective in IFIS. This is because the pupillary margin remains elastic, and the pupil immediately snaps back to its original size following attempts of stretching it.

Partial-thickness iris sphincter cuts made with microscissors is not a very common pupil-enlargement technique nowadays. It requires multiple maneuvers of the instrument inserted through the main incision or paracentesis inside the anterior chamber, which may result in corneal endothelial damage. Other disadvantages are similar to the stretching method (eg, bleeding and atonic pupil).

Several pupil-expansion devices for intraoperative use are available. Flexible plastic iris hooks are probably one of the most used devices worldwide. Traditionally, four hooks are introduced through evenly spaced 1.0-mm corneal incisions (Figure 21-2). The diamond-shaped configuration of the iris hooks is based on the placement of one of the hooks under the main phaco incision. This improves lens access by orienting the phaco needle movements along the square diagonal, which can be especially helpful in IFIS. It should be emphasized that iris hooks are the only devices that can help in cases with both a small pupil and zonular weakness. Use of the hooks allows the surgeon to temporarily fixate the capsular bag to the limbus, simultaneously stabilizing the capsular bag and enlarging the pupil aperture.

In contrast to iris hooks, one of the most attractive benefits of the mechanical pupil expanders or rings is the ability to avoid multiple additional incisions in the eye. The expansion ring is introduced and removed through the main phaco incision. Several pupil rings are currently available, including Perfect Pupil (Milvella), Morcher Ring (Morcher GmbH), Siepser Ring, and Graether Pupil Expander (Eagle Vision).

Malyugin Ring

One of the relatively new pupil expanding devices is the Malyugin Ring (MicroSurgical Technology) (Figure 21-3).[1-3] This square-shaped device, made of 6-0 polypropylene, is based on the "paper-clip" principle of iris margin fixation, with the coils located at its 4 corners. In spite of the square configuration, after Malyugin Ring placement, the enlarged pupil has a rounded shape (Figure 21-4). This is because the iris is retracted at 8 points (4 coils and 4 central portions of the ring side).

The Malyugin Ring System (MicroSurgical Technology) consists of a presterilized, single-use holder containing the ring and the inserter. The latter is used to implant the device and retract

Figure 21-3. General view of the Malyugin Ring.

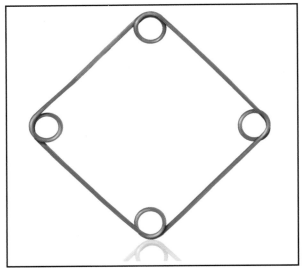

Figure 21-4. With a Malyugin Ring inserted, the pupil is retracted at 8 points (4 coils and 4 central portions of the ring side).

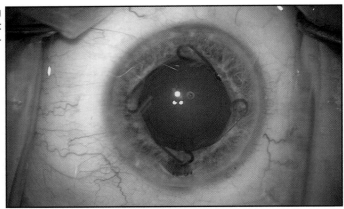

it from the eye. The surgical technique of Malyugin Ring implantation is as follows: after loading the ring into the inserter, its tip is introduced into the anterior chamber through the main incision. The tip of the inserter is positioned at the center of the anterior chamber. By pushing the thumb button, the ring is released from the tip forward, and the scroll is engaged with the distal iris (Figure 21-5A). The ring is slowly injected while simultaneously retracting the inserter (Figure 21-5B). Lateral scrolls emerge from the tube of the inserter and one (or both) of them simultaneously catch the iris margins. The proximal scroll is expelled from the cannula, and the inserter is moved until the injector hook is no longer holding the ring. The inserter is then withdrawn from the eye. If necessary, the Osher/Malyugin Ring manipulator (MicroSurgical Technology) (or Kuglen or Lester hook; Katena Products Inc) is used to engage the iris margin with the ring scrolls. In some cases, it is useful to disengage the proximal scroll from the injector with the help of a hook introduced through the paracentesis.

Phacoemulsification is then performed, followed by cortical material irrigation and aspiration and intraocular lens implantation. In small-pupil patients, phaco machine setting adjustments are also recommended. Fluidic parameters, such as irrigation bottle height, aspiration flow rate, and vacuum, should be lowered to decrease the fluid turbulence in the anterior chamber and to prevent the chance of iris aspiration into the phaco or irrigation/aspiration handpiece.

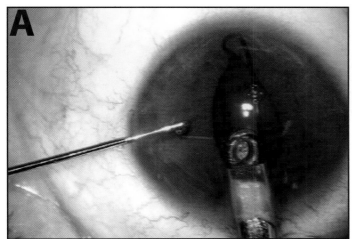

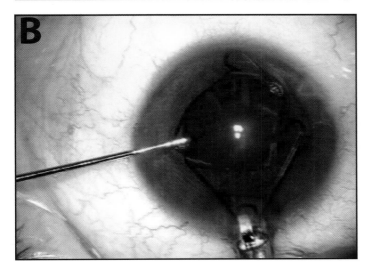

Figure 21-5. The Malyugin Ring injection steps. (A) The ring is released from the tip forward by pushing the thumb button and the scroll engages with the distal iris. (B) The ring is injected slowly while simultaneously retracting the inserter.

The Malyugin Ring is then removed from the eye in the reverse order. The inserter is introduced through the main incision, and its footplate is positioned under the proximal scroll. The inserter hook catches the proximal scroll and retracts the ring inside the inserter tube. To retract the ring completely inside the injector, it is often necessary to press with a side-port instrument on the lateral scrolls when they merge. With this maneuver, the surgeon can avoid catching the rim of the injector with the lateral scroll, which is located above, and subsequent twisting of the ring. After Malyugin Ring removal, the pupil constricts spontaneously (Figure 21-6). The procedure is completed with OVD removal and checking the self-sealing properties of the corneal wounds.

Patients with poorly dilated pupils are prone to a more intense postoperative inflammatory response due to ocular comorbidity and extra manipulations of the iris tissue. For this reason, one should consider closer follow-up, and intensive and prolonged pharmacotherapy combining steroids and nonsteroidal anti-inflammatory drugs.

Figure 21-6. After Malyugin Ring removal, the pupil constricts spontaneously.

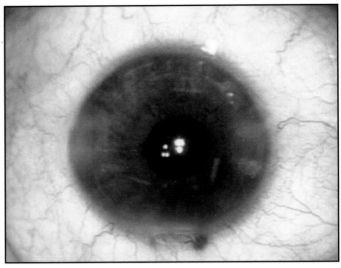

References

1. Malyugin B. Small pupil phaco surgery: a new technique. *Ann Ophthalmol (Skokie)*. 2007;39(3):185-193.
2. Chang DF. Use of Malyugin pupil expansion device for intraoperative floppy-iris syndrome: results in 30 consecutive cases. *J Cataract Refract Surg*. 2008;34(5):835–841.
3. Malyugin B. Review of surgical management of small pupils in cataract surgery. Use of the Malyugin Ring. *Techniques in Ophthalmology*. 2010;8(3):1-15.

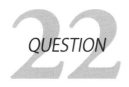

WHAT SHOULD I DO IF THE CHAMBER IS SO SHALLOW THAT IT DOES NOT DEEPEN MUCH WITH VISCOELASTIC?

Lisa Brothers Arbisser, MD

Preventing complications is the best strategy for surgery. Recognize the crowded anterior chambered eye preoperatively. These occur more commonly in the Asian population and short hyperopic and, especially, nanophthalmic eyes. The slit-lamp examination raises suspicion, confirmed by the IOLMaster (Carl Zeiss Meditec Inc), when the anterior chamber depth measurement is usually less than 2.5 mm. Shallow chambers require gonioscopy to confirm closeable angles, which are treated with laser peripheral iridotomy prior to cataract surgery. In cases of borderline gonioscopy, preoperatively measure the intraocular pressure after tropicamide-only dilation to diagnose, reverse, and treat relative angle closure.

With the use of 0.25 g per kg of Mannitol intravenous push 15 minutes prior to surgery in shallow-chambered eyes, even postperipheral iridotomy is advisable. Consider digital massage to lower the vitreous pressure. In eyes with plateau iris, consider intracameral dilation with lidocaine and epinephrine, without preoperative dilation, to avoid any chance of early pupillary block when the patient comes to the operating table.

How to Maintain the Chamber

If at any time during the procedure the chamber cannot be maintained, despite the details elaborated herein, it may be necessary to consider a dry vitreous tap through the pars plana for the best outcome. This is rarely required; however, it is advisable to keep vitrectomy equipment, a 78-diopter lens and indirect ophthalmoscope, available.

The corneal incision should not be too peripheral and should fit the phaco tip snugly. The paracentesis should be 0.5 mm to maintain a closed chamber during lens removal. When making the incision, closely monitor iris movement toward the internal Descemet's membrane to prevent full prolapse into the tunnel. Never stuff a prolapsed iris back into the wound or it becomes more floppy and diaphanous. Instead, decompress the chamber through the paracentesis, allowing the iris to reposit.

Then, create space for surgery with the use of a more viscous or highly retentive ophthalmic viscosurgical device (OVD). I prefer a soft-shell technique,[1] with Viscoat (Alcon Laboratories) against the endothelium and Healon GV OVD (Abbott Medical Optics Inc) below to flatten the capsule dome. Healon5 (Abbott Medical Optics Inc) can easily overdeepen the chamber, raising pressure precipitously and promoting iris prolapse. Assuming that it is possible to deepen the chamber for capsulorrhexis adequately, the key step for a successful outcome, I recommend an intraocular or slim opening Utrata Capsulorrhexis Forceps (Medetz Surgical Instruments) to minimize any chance of chamber loss during the capsule manipulation. It is equally important to maintain control of the vector, directed centripetally, which cannot be as reliably managed with a needle rhexis technique. A conservatively sized rhexis with subsequent enlargement at the case's conclusion makes it less likely for the rhexis to extend peripherally.

Gentle, minimal-volume, and multidirectional hydrodissection facilitates freeing the nucleus, which is often too large to rotate well. Mindfulness of volume and simultaneous decompression of the bag, with subtle pressure on the posterior scleral lip and central nucleus, will avoid the catastrophe of posterior capsule rupture due to tamponade that can otherwise occur.

Filling the chamber with more dispersive OVD prior to entry with the phaco tip restores the endothelial shield that is partially lost during hydrodissection, which is especially critical in a shallow chambered eye, and prevents stripping of Descemet's membrane on entry. Consciously establish flow in foot-position 2 prior to engaging ultrasound in an OVD-filled environment to avoid wound burn. A vertical phaco-chop technique allows the tip to remain in the safe zone within the rhexis and the often-small pupil in these cases. Remove one small pie wedge of nucleus after the main central chop facilitates rotation of the nucleus. Chop the remainder into small sections before removing it so that most of the phaco energy is dispersed at the iris plane or below. Do not bring a large piece of the nucleus into the anterior chamber. A noncontinuous ultrasound delivery strategy is always desirable.

Short eyes are always prone to retrodirected fluid syndrome and to suprachoroidal hemorrhage. These risks are minimized by maintaining a normotensive eye as much as possible and always preventing collapse of the anterior chamber. Supporting the chamber by exchanging the second-hand instrument for balanced salt solution in a 3-mL syringe with a 26-gauge cannula (so there is irrigation through the side port when withdrawing the phaco or aspiration tip) facilitates this goal. After the nucleus is gone, these eyes will often behave in a more normal fashion, although every step until completion requires attention to detail.

As previously mentioned, any time the chamber is too shallow or the eye is too firm to proceed, consider a dry pars plana vitreous tap. If the eye suddenly hardens, employ a 78-diopter lens with the microscope or sterile-technique indirect ophthalmoscopy prior to a sclerotomy to rule out hemorrhage.

If topical anesthesia is used, the patient will require a subconjunctival bleb of lidocaine with epinephrine to be injected with a sharp 30-gauge needle over the quadrant where the sclerotomy will be performed, for comfort and hemostasis.

Historically, a sharp needle on a simple syringe through the pars plana was used to remove vitreous, assuming the needle will find a pocket of liquid vitreous. Unfortunately, this is a hit-or-miss method that flirts with the catastrophe of vitreous traction, retinal tear, and detachment; therefore, it is strongly discouraged. The safer option is to use automated vitrectomy.[2,3]

The vitrector is set to cut before vacuum begins. Remove the irrigation sleeve, if present, so the vitrector needle is bare, and pinch the irrigation line shut. Employ the highest cut rate available. The flow rate is set to 20 g for a 20-g or 15 g for 23-g vitrector, which is the usual default. The vacuum is set to 150 mm Hg for 20 g and 350 mm Hg for 23 g, which is the lower end of the

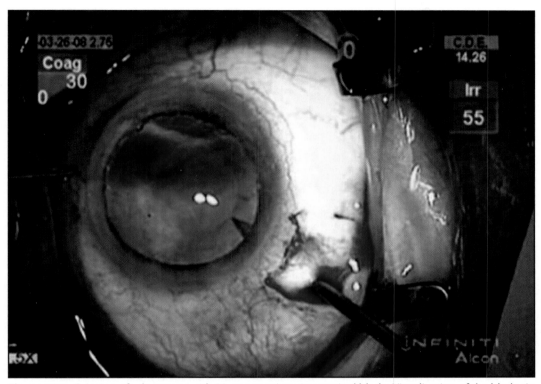

Figure 22-1. Creation of sclerotomy with 20-gauge microvitreoretinal blade. Visualization of the blade tip within the pupillary space confirms complete entry.

default linear setting. I recommend the vacuum be set as nonlinear or fixed. This allows surgeons lacking vitrectomy experience to have the same safe level of vacuum throughout foot-position 3.

I prefer a straight microvitreoretinal blade and do not recommend a trocar system, which requires more entrance pressure and increases the risk of tagging the posterior capsule. Create a small peritomy in the quadrant convenient to the surgeon's dominant hand. Use a caliper to measure 3.5 mm posterior to the limbus. Avoid penetrating vessels, or use a spot of eraser-tip cautery. Enter perpendicular to the sclera, and aim toward the optic nerve. Mindful that lens thickness in small eyes is greater than in average globes, maintain an acute angle to avoid cutting the posterior capsule. Ideally, visualize the tip of the blade in the pupil to confirm complete entry (Figure 22-1). If there is no view due to a dense cataract, it is prudent to measure 10 mm from the tip of the vitrector and make a scratch or mark along the shaft so that on entry the vitrector will not be accidentally inserted too deeply beyond the center of the pupil. Prior to entry, the vitrector port is turned so that the opening will be sideways (more inferior facing than superior) and it won't suck up the posterior capsule. The globe is best stabilized by a cellulose sponge with the tip cut off, held in the nondominant hand. The vitrector is inserted, with the irrigation pinched off outside the eye. Just after insertion, the foot pedal is depressed to foot-position 2 to activate cutting without vacuum whenever moving through vitreous to avoid traction. After the vitrector is in place in the middle of the pupil behind the lens, pointing backwards or sideways, the pedal is depressed to the metal in foot-position 3 (vacuum will never exceed the panel setting). The cellulose sponge in the nondominant hand is in position to assess the softening of the globe, as only a few seconds of vitrector action will accomplish the goal of removing approximately 0.2 cc of vitreous. This allows the anterior chamber to be deepened for safe cataract surgery. Removing more vitreous than

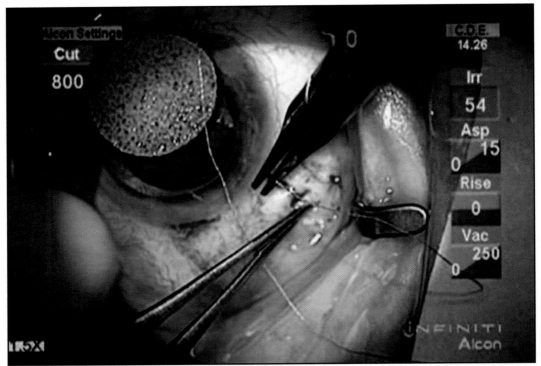

Figure 22-2. Suturing of sclerotomy. An "X" or double-bite mattress 8-0 Vicryl suture can be used to close the incision.

necessary can lead to a challenging surgery with an abnormally deep chamber and soft eye that risks suprachoroidal hemorrhage.

When an endpoint is likely reached, the anterior chamber is filled with OVD through the paracentesis to a normotensive point and a normal or slightly shallow depth by exchanging the cellulose sponge in the nondominant hand for the OVD syringe, while holding the vitrector stable inside the eye, thereby controlling movement of the eye during this manipulation. If more space is needed, a bit more vitreous can be removed. When ideal, the vitrector is retracted toward the sclerotomy in foot-position 2 (cutting without vacuum) to avoid dragging vitreous and causing traction that can lead to retinal tear.

On exiting the sclera, a scleral plug is a nice luxury so that the sclerotomy can be easily reentered if needed; otherwise, the sclerotomy must be closed, so the globe once again is whole, to proceed with surgery. If any vitreous remains between the lips of the sclerotomy, the vitrector can be used at the surface of the sclera over the incision to sever any strands. An "X" or double-bite mattress 8-0 Vicryl suture can be tied temporarily with a bowknot if a plug is not available (Figure 22-2). The case should now proceed normally.

References

1. Tarongoy P, Ho CL, Walton DS. Angle-closure glaucoma: the role of the lens in the pathogenesis, prevention, and treatment. *Surv Ophthalmol*. 2009;54(2):211-225.
2. Mackool RJ. Pars plana vitreous tap for phacoemulsification in the crowded eye. *J Cataract Refract Surg*. 2002;28(4):572-573.
3. Chang DF. Pars plana vitreous tap for phacoemulsification in the crowded eye. *J Cataract Refract Surg*. 2001;27(12):1911-1914.

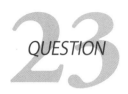

My Capsulorrhexis Is Heading Out Peripherally. How Should I Proceed, and What Should I Do if it Tears Radially?

Brian Little, MA, DO, FHEA, FRCS, FRCOphth

A radialized tear of the capsulorrhexis is a disappointing way to start any cataract operation. The good news is that if you stop before it has gone too far out and into the zonules, with a little ingenuity and know-how, it is usually retrievable.

It is probably true to say that, in an ideal world, every capsulorrhexis tear-out can be avoided, given enough care and attention. I really do believe that, in principle, we should adopt a zero-tolerance attitude toward this complication, which means setting the bar high from the start. In doing so, we establish a counsel of perfection that is a good starting point from which to set out. Prevention is a lot easier than retrieval.

Common Causes of Radial Tear-Out

Overwhelmingly, the most common cause of a radial tear-out is allowing the chamber to shallow due to progressive loss of viscoelastic through the main wound. That tear-outs keep happening with the same incidence for this same reason is testimonial to the fact that we tend to focus too hard on what is happening at the point of the tear and not enough on what is happening to the chamber depth. Chamber swallowing can be minimized by habitually refilling with ophthalmic viscosurgical device (OVD) routinely after every 90 to 120 degrees of the rhexis. This is a worthwhile habit to get into early on, as it teaches the surgeon to appreciate the large volume of OVD that rapidly leaves the eye in the early stages of the rhexis.

The other reason that the rhexis continues to tear out once it starts is simply that we allow it to do so. By this, I mean that, despite our noticing that it is starting to creep out, we are not very good at stopping immediately and sorting it out. We tend to put on blinders, keep pushing ahead, deny there is a problem, and continue to pull the flap until the tear goes out further, until we are forced to stop. Instead of stopping when we first notice a potential problem, we tend to continue

Figure 23-1. A radialized rhexis is noted inferiorly.

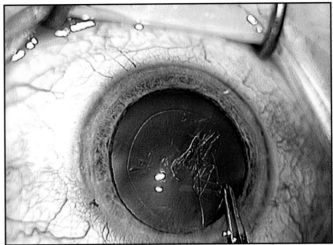

Figure 23-2. Anterior chamber is overfilled with OVD, to tamponade and flatten the anterior lens capsule and help minimize further peripheral migration of the tear.

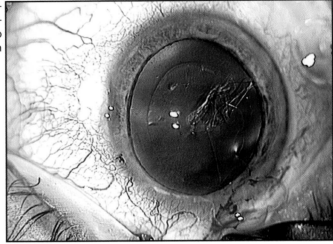

until we have a definite problem and then have no choice but to stop. We need to learn the self-discipline to stop at the first sign of trouble.

If, despite your best efforts, the rhexis has radialized (Figure 23-1), then you should stop immediately and resist the temptation to give it the final "pull of hope," usually done with eyes closed, teeth clenched, and accompanied by a tachycardia. It never works. Instead, just come out and overfill the chamber with OVD, so to tamponade and flatten the anterior lens capsule and help minimize further peripheral migration of the tear (Figure 23-2). You are now ready to attempt retrieval of the tear.

Retrieval of the Tear

In principle, you have to unfold the flap, grab it near the root of the tear, pull it back first circumferentially and then centrally to redirect the tear inward.[1] The devil, as ever, is in the detail,

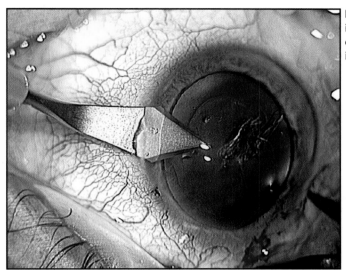

Figure 23-3. A second stab incision is made at a position that allows the optimal angle of approach for applying traction on the capsular flap.

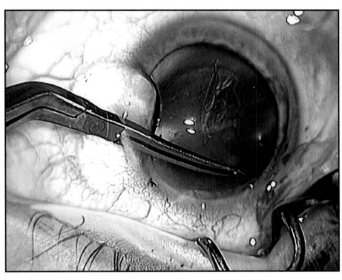

Figure 23-4. Grasp the flap as near to the root of the tear as is practically possible and apply traction in the horizontal plane of the capsule. Do not lift forward.

and there are 9 important points that will maximize your chances of success and avoid disappointment. They are as follows:

1. Completely fill the chamber with viscoelastic before any attempt at retrieval.

2. If necessary, make a second stab incision at the position that allows the optimal angle of approach for applying traction (Figure 23-3).

3. Unfold the flap of the anterior capsule and flatten it against the lens (visco-manipulation).

4. If visibility is compromised, then have a low threshold for painting trypan blue onto the anterior capsule underneath the OVD to visualize the edges of the tear.

5. Refill the chamber immediately before attempting retrieval.

6. Use rhexis forceps only. Do not attempt this procedure with a needle. The directional control is inadequate, and you are likely to puncture or tear the flap with the force required.

7. Grasp the flap as near to the root of the tear as is practically possible (Figure 23-4).

Figure 23-5. The initial pull should be circumferentially backwards. While holding the flap in tension, pull more centrally to initiate the tear.

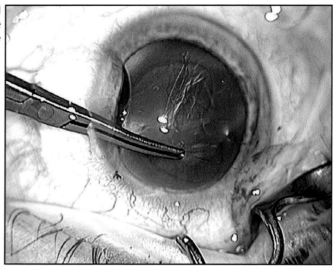

Figure 23-6. Centrally directed tear propagates toward the center and avoids further radialization of the anterior capsular tear.

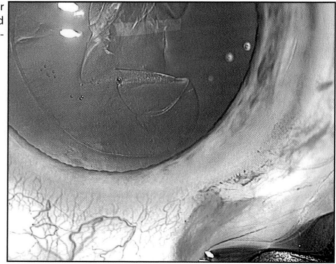

8. Apply traction in the horizontal plane of the capsule, and do not lift forward.

9. The initial pull should be circumferentially backwards and, while holding the flap in tension, pull more centrally to initiate the tear, which will then propagate toward the center (Figures 23-5 and 23-6).

The biggest mystery is to know how much force can be applied safely. The answer is as much as you feel safe using, which gets clearer as you become more experienced. If it will not tear, and the whole lens is being pulled centrally, then there is a risk that you will get a wraparound tear, in which case you should stop and abandon it to complete the rhexis, either from the other direction or make a relieving tangential cut in the edge of the flap and continue in the same direction.

Using the outlined principles, I have not (yet) had one wraparound tear and have had to abandon only a handful of tears.

The technique can be viewed at the following online video, "Little Technique on Lumera" at http://www.youtube.com/watch?v=6xEnMPBaNPM.

Conclusion

Naturally you will feel very anxious during your first attempt at this technique. Once you have succeeded, your confidence will increase exponentially, and you will rapidly overcome your hesitancy and enjoy the satisfaction of its success.

Reference

1. Little BC, Smith JH, Packer M. Little capsulorrhexis tear-out rescue. *J Cataract Refract Surg.* 2006;32(9):1420-1422.

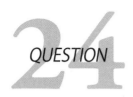

FOLLOWING HYDRODISSECTION, THE IRIS IS PROLAPSING AND THE GLOBE IS VERY FIRM. HOW SHOULD I PROCEED?

Mark Packer, MD, FACS, CPI

Injection of excessive hydrodissection fluid has most likely precipitated the sudden increase in pressure and the concomitant ejection of iris tissue. A bulging anterior lens surface accompanied by a widened capsulotomy diameter confirms the most likely mechanism: excess fluid trapped inside the lens capsule. (Figures 24-1 through 24-5 demonstrate the proper method of cortical cleaving hydrodissection. Performing each step as described will help to avoid iris prolapse and other problems.)[1] Forward movement of the lens and distention of the capsule has displaced viscoelastic material in the posterior chamber, pushing the iris out of the incision. The iris prolapse may be exacerbated by a suboptimal surgical technique, such as a relatively short, excessively wide, or posteriorly placed incision. The presence of risk factors for intraoperative floppy iris syndrome (ie, systemic alpha receptor antagonist medications) also may predispose toward iris prolapse.[2]

Releasing the Fluid

Decompression of the capsule is achieved by using the hydrodissection cannula through a paracentesis port to push the lens nucleus posteriorly. The fluid trapped between the lens and the posterior capsule is forced to flow anteriorly around the equator of the lens. As the fluid is released, the capsulotomy diameter narrows, and the lens returns to its natural position. Release of fluid and viscoelastic material from the anterior chamber is achieved by repeatedly pushing on the posterior lip of the paracentesis with the edge of the cannula.

Figure 24-1. The anterior capsule is tented up with a 26-gauge cannula to create space between the capsule and the cortex to inject balanced salt solution.

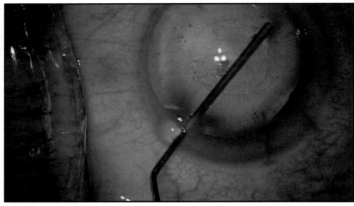

Figure 24-2. Fluid is injected firmly under the capsule and, as the fluid wave begins to spread posteriorly, the lip of the incision is depressed with the cannula to allow viscoelastic to exit.

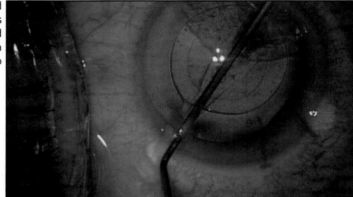

Figure 24-3. As the fluid wave completes its transit of the posterior capsule, the lens bulges anteriorly and the capsulorrhexis opening enlarges due to increased pressure from trapped hydrodissection fluid between the cortex and the posterior capsule. The pressure in the eye is at maximum, and a large amount of viscoelastic flows out of the incisions. This is the moment of greatest risk of overpressurization, leading to iris prolapse.

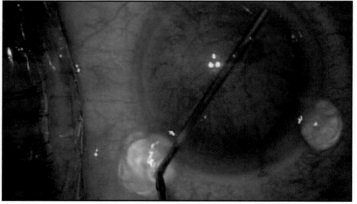

Reposing the Iris

After the intraocular pressure is reduced, the iris may be reposited. Directly pushing on the iris with an instrument tends to damage it further, causing release of pigment and the creation of an iridotomy. A better method involves sweeping the iris into the eye from a side-port incision with the side of a cannula. When the iris is back inside the anterior chamber, a dispersive viscoelastic

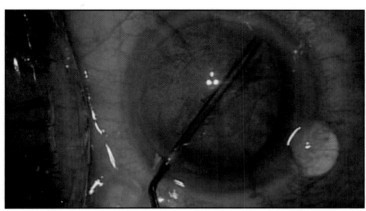

Figure 24-4. The side of the cannula is used to depress the lens firmly, decompressing the capsule and pushing the trapped fluid anteriorly around the equator of the lens. The capsulorrhexis opening returns to its former size, and the pressure in the eye is relieved.

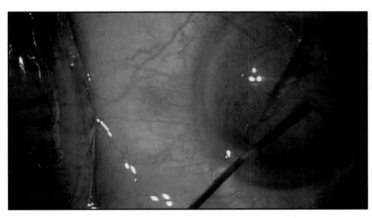

Figure 24-5. The lens is now ready for rotation. The mark of the cannula on the anterior lens surface indicates the amount of pressure that was used to decompress the capsule.

agent may be injected directly above it at the location of prolapse, effectively pushing the iris tissue posteriorly.

Rotation of the Lens

Rotation of the lens may now be accomplished, preferably without further hydrodissection, and hydrodelineation may be carried out in standard gentle fashion.[3] During phacoemulsification, the presence of the tip in the incision will preclude further iris prolapse; however, the damaged iris tissue is often flaccid and prone to aspiration and shredding. Care should be taken to avoid touching the iris with the phaco tip. In case of severe flaccidity, iris hooks placed to either side of the incision may be used. It is not advisable to attempt placement of a pupil ring at this stage of the procedure due to the potential for further damage to the iris and incarceration of the capsulotomy edge in the ring.

Consideration should be given to the status of the lens capsule and zonular fibers if any step of this recovery procedure does not produce the desired result. Generally, rupture of the posterior capsule during hydrodissection results in sudden deepening of the anterior chamber and descent of the nucleus, rather than shallowing and iris prolapse. However, injection of hydrodissection fluid through a capsular rent or through the zonular fibers directly into the vitreous space will increase posterior pressure, shallow the anterior chamber, and cause iris prolapse. If pushing the lens nucleus posteriorly does not result in the expected release of fluid, then hydration of the vitreous is the likely problem. Intravenous mannitol may be administered,[4] or a pars plana vitreous tap or limited vitrectomy may be performed.[5]

Other Causes of Increased Intraocular Pressure and Iris Prolapse

Less likely mechanisms of increased intraocular pressure (IOP) and iris prolapse should be considered in the complete differential diagnosis. External pressure on the eye from coughing, straining, or eyelid squeezing on the part of an anxious patient may produce iris prolapse, but it will not result in a firm eye. Ask the patient whether he or she is comfortable, provide a throat lozenge to the patient under the drapes, administer additional intravenous medication such as midazolam, or consider performing a lid block.[6]

Malposition of the eyelid speculum, particularly if a blade is not securely seated in the fornix and the eyelid is inverted, puts persistent pressure on the eye and may cause iris prolapse and a firm eye. A retrobulbar hemorrhage, very unlikely with topical anesthesia, may dramatically increase IOP. In the presence of sudden onset of proptosis, the surgeon should perform a lateral canthotomy and cantholysis.[7]

Intraocular pressure rises precipitously in the presence of a suprachoroidal hemorrhage, resulting in severe pain, loss of the red reflex, shallowing of the anterior chamber, iris prolapse, and potential expulsion of the lens, vitreous, and retina. Initial management is direct tamponade and rapid wound closure.[8] Viscoelastic agents may help to deepen the anterior chamber. Excision of prolapsed tissue may be necessary. Drainage through posterior sclerostomies may be needed to relieve pressure and permit wound closure.

Conclusion

There are a variety of causes of increased IOP and iris prolapse at the time of surgery. Correctly identifying the cause will allow the surgeon to quickly remedy the situation and facilitate a good outcome.

References

1. Fine IH. Cortical cleaving hydrodissection. *J Cataract Refract Surg.* 1992;18(5):508-512.
2. Goseki T, Ishikawa H, Ogasawara S, et al. Effects of tamsulosin and silodosin on isolated albino and pigmented rabbit iris dilators: possible mechanism of intraoperative floppy-iris syndrome. *J Cataract Refract Surg.* 2012;38(9):1643-1649.
3. Fine IH, Hoffman RS, Packer M. Hydrodissection and hydrodelineation. In Steinert V, ed. *Cataract Surgery.* 3rd ed. Philadelphia, PA: Elsevier; 2012:173-178.
4. O'Keeffe M, Nabil M. The use of mannitol in intraocular surgery. *Ophthalmic Surg.* 1983;14(1):55-56.
5. Chalam KV, Gupta SK, Agarwal S, Shah VA. Sutureless limited vitrectomy for positive vitreous pressure in cataract surgery. *Ophthalmic Surg Lasers Imaging.* 2005;36(6):518-522.
6. Schimek F, Fahle M. Techniques of facial nerve block. *Br J Ophthalmol.* 1995;79(2):166-173.
7. Ballard SR, Enzenauer RW, O'Donnell T, et al. Emergency lateral canthotomy and cantholysis: a simple procedure to preserve vision from sight threatening orbital hemorrhage. *J Spec Oper Med.* 2009;9(3):26-32.
8. Ling R, Cole M, James C, et al. Suprachoroidal haemorrhage complicating cataract surgery in the UK: epidemiology, clinical features, management, and outcomes. *Br J Ophthalmol.* 2004;88(4):478-480.

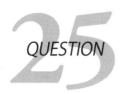

Despite Attempting Hydrodissection, I Cannot Rotate the Nucleus. How Should I Proceed?

William J. Fishkind, MD, FACS

The hydrosteps consist of hydrodissection and hydrodelineation. To describe the management of the inability to achieve nuclear rotation after hydrodissection, I will first clarify how to perform cortical-cleaving hydrodissection properly.

Cortical-Cleaving Hydrodissection

In cortical-cleaving hydrodissection,[1,2] I prefer a standard 27-gauge cannula attached to a 3-cc syringe filled with balanced salt solution (BSS). However, any cannula designed for this function is placed just superior to the anterior capsular remnant, then withdrawn slightly and dropped just below the anterior capsule. The tip is advanced and elevated under the anterior capsule until it is halfway between the anterior capsular rim and the capsular-bag equator. This assures a peripheral position between the cortex and anterior capsule. The tip of the cannula is elevated, tenting the anterior capsule.

A steady, firm stream of BSS is then injected. The stream of BSS passes both anteriorly toward the capsulorrhexis edge, as well as around the proximate equator, behind the posterior pole of the cataract, and around to the opposite equator and into the anterior chamber. Slight depression of the shaft of the cannula against the posterior lip of the incision during fluid injection allows excess fluid to pass out of the incision, thereby reducing excessive pressure in the anterior chamber. This is especially important if a dispersive ophthalmic viscosurgical device (OVD) is used. The endpoint of fluid injection is the visualization of the cataract floating anteriorly. Gentle posterior pressure on the cataract will effectively push fluid sequestered behind the nucleus around the equator (Figure 25-1).

The hydrodissection should be performed first on one side of the cataract and then again in a location 180 degrees opposite. If performed effectively, the cortex is separated, or cleaved, from

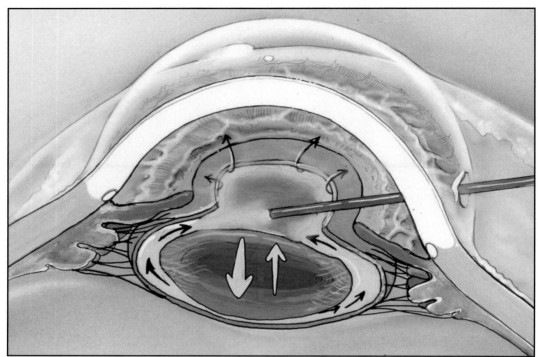

Figure 25-1. Illustration of fluid surrounding the nucleus and cortex peripherally separating cortex from capsular bag. The thin white arrow indicates the lens floating anteriorly due to hydrostatic pressure from fluid trapped behind the cataract. The wide white arrow indicates downward pressure from the cannula to squeeze fluid around the cataract, creating a fluid dissection of cortex from the capsular bag. The black arrows indicate the flow of fluid from behind the cataract, around the equator, and out the anterior capsular opening. (From Fishkind WJ, ed. *Complications in Phacoemulsification: Avoidance, Recognition, and Management*. New York, NY: Thieme Medical Publishers; 2002. Reprinted with permission.)

the capsule, allowing free rotation of the endonucleus, epinucleus, and cortex as a unit within the capsular bag. This will lyse all nuclear, cortical, and capsular bag connections (Figure 25-2).

Standard Hydrodissection

Standard hydrodissection is performed in a similar manner, except the cannula is placed within the substance of the cortex. This produces a cleavage plane within the cortex. Consequently, part of the cortex remains adherent to the capsular bag and part to the endonucleus.

Hydrodelineation

Immediately following hydrodissection, the same cannula is moved to the paracentral zone of the nucleus and embedded within the nuclear substance. The cannula tip is moved to and fro to create a track within the nuclear material. Balanced salt solution is then injected slowly into the bulk of the nucleus. The BSS will find the surgical plane at the junction of the epinucleus and

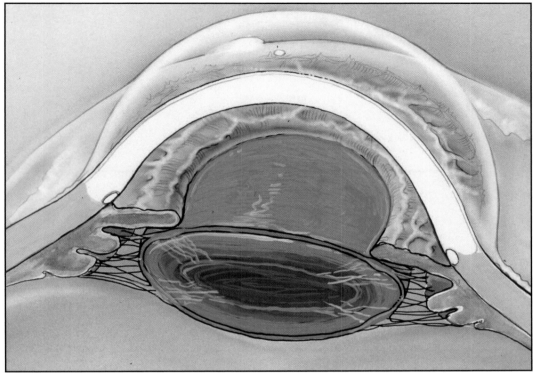

Figure 25-2. Illustration of the nuclear, cortical, and capsular-bag connections, which must be lysed to allow unrestrained rotation of the cataract. (From Fishkind WJ, ed. *Complications in Phacoemulsification: Avoidance, Recognition, and Management.* New York, NY: Thieme Medical Publishers; 2002. Reprinted with permission.)

endonucleus and divide them. Even after adequate hydrodelineation, the endonucleus will not rotate independently of adjacent epinucleus and cortex.

Hydrodelineation is necessary to perform those phaco procedures requiring lens disassembly methodology (ie, phaco-chop).

Why Perform Cortical-Cleaving Hydrodissection?

There are several reasons to switch from conventional hydrodissection to cortical-cleaving hydrodissection. The latter technique is performed more peripherally to cleave cortex from the capsular bag. The surgeon then can separate the endonucleus from the epinucleus and cortex via hydrodelineation. These two actions permit a 2-procedure phacoemulsification, with removal of the endonucleus initially, then the epinucleus and adherent cortex. As the cataract becomes more nuclear mature, the epinucleus becomes increasingly important to function as a protective shell. It will prevent sharp fragments of nucleus from tearing the posterior capsule, especially if a surge should occur. After the endonucleus is emulsified, the cataract will lose its rigidity. The cortical shell can be elevated easily to the plane of the iris for emulsification, using lower-power and vacuum settings to minimize surge. The lysis of cortical-bag connections allows more complete cortical removal during phaco. This serves to minimize irrigation and aspiration time, and relieves stress to the zonules and ciliary body during irrigation and aspiration.

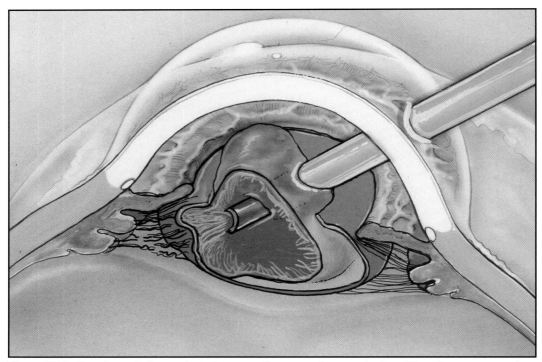

Figure 25-3. The phaco tip has aspirated cortex adherent to the capsular bag. The adherent cortex does not separate from the bag. Pulling on the endonucleus to rotate it or aspirating endonucleus will result in breaking adjacent zonules. (From Fishkind WJ, ed. *Complications in Phacoemulsification: Avoidance, Recognition, and Management.* New York, NY: Thieme Medical Publishers; 2002. Reprinted with permission.)

In the presence of a torn posterior capsule, cortical-cleaving hydrodissection facilitates the removal of cortex during irrigation and aspiration without enlarging the tear, as the cortex is not adherent to the capsular bag. If the patient's zonules are weak, cortical-cleaving hydrodissection eases the removal of the epinucleus and cortex, thus avoiding tearing more zonules and disrupting the capsular bag.

Adherent Epinucleus and Cortex

The previously mentioned steps should ensure a freely rotating nucleus 95% of the time. If the nucleus does not turn freely, then the hydrodissection was incomplete, and the surgeon should repeat the procedure. In fact, hydrodissection can be performed at any time; therefore, the phaco can be interrupted after the initial chop in vertical chopping or grove and crack in stop and chop, and hydrodissection can be repeated. The crack in the nucleus presents an egress path for BSS. This will generate space for a natural fluid path under and around the heminucleus, completing the hydrodissection. Occasionally, with a small amount of OVD to maintain the anterior chamber and working against the counter pressure of the vitreous, two instruments can be introduced to tire iron the nucleus and free it from the capsular bag.[3] If the nucleus does not rotate freely, divide-and-conquer and horizontal chopping are contraindicated. The rotational maneuvers necessary for divide-and-conquer may result in stressed and torn zonules or a tear in the capsular bag (Figure 25-3).

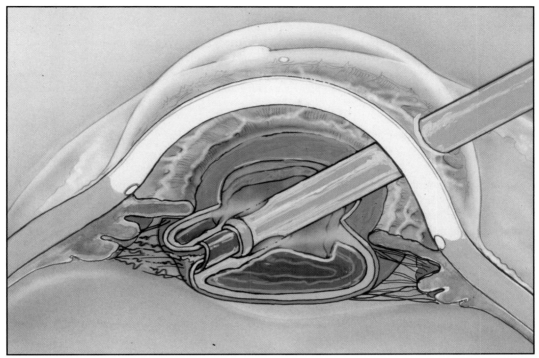

Figure 25-4. With continued aspiration, the equatorial capsular bag will be engaged and torn. (From Fishkind WJ, ed. *Complications in Phacoemulsification: Avoidance, Recognition, and Management.* New York, NY: Thieme Medical Publishers; 2002. Reprinted with permission.)

Trying to place the chopper around the equator of the lens when it is still attached to the capsular bag may have a similar result.

If repeated and full hydrodissection is impossible, the surgeon must exercise greater care during phacoemulsification, so as not to stress the zonules or approach the equatorial cortical material too closely, and phaco through the equatorial bag (Figure 25-4). If complete hydrodissection appears impossible and the nucleus will not freely rotate, then, as previously described, vertical chopping is the technique of choice. Eventually, enough endonucleus will be removed so that the remaining endonucleus and cortex will become mobile. Remember to use caution in this situation, because an immobile nucleus may indicate an occult tear in the capsular bag or weak zonules.

Intentional Incomplete Hydrodissection

Occasionally, the conscious decision not to complete a hydrodissection is indicated. A nick in the anterior capsule or a discontinuous capsulorrhexis (eg, one that extended toward the equator and had to be finished from the other side) are good reasons not to complete hydrodissection. The addition of too much fluid will cause a capsular tear to extend to the equator, or worse, into the posterior capsule. Another reason surgeons might hesitate to complete hydrodissection is poor visualization due to a small pupil. In addition, some might forego complete dissection in cases of preexisting weak zonules caused by earlier zonular trauma, zonular tears, or pseudoexfoliation. Although it is difficult to hydrodissect and fully rotate the nucleus in these cases, I believe they actually require extra hydrodissection. A Malyugin Ring (MicroSurgical Technology Inc),

MacKool capsular bag support hooks (Bausch & Lomb Inc), Cionni or Henderson capsular tension rings (FCI Ophthalmics), or Ahmed capsular ring segments (FCI Ophthalmics) permit enhanced outcomes for complete hydrodissection. If the surgeon can continue to work carefully with multiple small hydrodissections until the nucleus is completely free within the capsular bag, then emulsifying the endonucleus, epinucleus, and cortex will be easier and less likely to damage the zonules further. Finally, posterior polar cataract calls for special hydrodissection maneuvers that are addressed in Chapter 38.

Conclusion

Cortical-cleaving hydrodissection and hydrodelineation occur early in the continuum of cataract surgery. Performed carefully, successful completion leads to an easier surgical procedure. Encountering adherent nucleus or cortex that will not rotate is a salvageable problem. Recognition and careful further hydrodissection, or performance of vertical chopping, will generally save the procedure.

References

1. Fishkind WJ. *Complications in Phacoemulsification: Avoidance, Recognition, and Management*. New York, NY: Thieme Medical Publishers; 2002.
2. Fine IH. Cortical cleaving hydrodissection. *J Cataract Refract Surg*. 1992;18(5):508-512.
3. Chang DF. *Phaco Chop: Mastering Techniques, Optimizing Technology, and Avoiding Complications*. Thorofare, NJ: SLACK Incorporated; 2013.

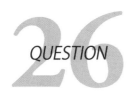

I Usually Perform Divide-and-Conquer Phacoemulsification. How Can I Incorporate Chopping Into My Technique?

Randall J. Olson, MD

Divide-and-conquer phacoemulsification, a tried-and-true procedure, represents most US and Canadian cataract surgeries. Increasingly, however, people have moved toward chopping techniques.[1] Those who favor the divide-and-conquer method cite its simplicity and effectiveness; yet, there remain compelling reasons for changing technique.

Advantages of chopping include efficiency and safety. Regarding efficiency, what encourages ultrasound use in other approaches, such as making grooves, is rapidly achieved through mechanical chopping.[2] Rather than taking time to create troughs or remove large pieces of the nucleus, it is split into smaller fragments, so ultrasound use becomes minimal. I use ultrasound for aspiration, for a fraction of the time that otherwise is necessary. An advantage of decreased ultrasound use is a decreased incidence of wound burns.[3]

Safety Concerns Related to Ultrasound

Safety concerns also are relevant to ultrasound risk. If the phaco tip breaks a capsule, usually ultrasound is on simultaneously, as aspiration alone will not cause breakage.[4] If procedures done using ultrasound are far from the cornea, iris, and capsule, difficulties with these tissues are less likely. Safety is hard to show when operating on straightforward cataracts, but it becomes noticeable in patients with a marginal cornea; a hard cataract, where mechanical forces are safer than using prolonged ultrasound; weak zonules; or complicated cases such as trauma with zonular dehiscence or small pupils.

Figure 26-1. The first horizontal chop is completed, and the nucleus is cleaved into heminuclei. Notice the separation both by the red reflex and the depth of the chopper and phaco tip into the nucleus. The usual reason this fails for beginners is due to not going deep enough with both instruments, especially the chopper. Horizontal choppers are made to be safe near the capsule.

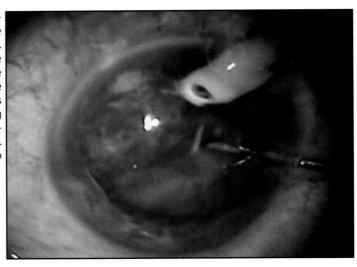

Chop Variations

Considering these potential advantages, why don't divide-and-conquer surgeons convert to chop? The deterrent is the clear learning curve, which is often scary due to complete and slightly difficult dependence on always using both hands. Although this is an initial barrier, beginners with patience can master the technique. I know no one who goes back to divide-and-conquer after realizing the advantages of chop.

Understanding the variations, which have advantages and disadvantages, is important.

Classical horizontal chop, outlined by Nagahara, involves impaling the nucleus with the phacoemulsification tip and using the second instrument to go around the pole of the nucleus and pull it toward the tip, separating the nucleus in half (Figure 26-1).[5] Because motions are largely horizontal, with the patient recumbent, we call this horizontal chopping.

Another approach is vertical chop, also known as quick chop. With the nucleus impaled, a thinner and slightly sharper instrument used to penetrate into the nucleus is introduced and then is separated from the tip, causing vertical shearing (Figures 26-2 and 26-3). It is not necessary to go underneath the pupil, and the tip is always visible. Other advantages concern the nucleus type encountered; often, a cleaner cut completely through the posterior plate is achieved.

Most surgeons evolve with some variation of the 2 techniques because, at times, one has distinct advantages over the other. A newer variation, prechop, uses instrumentation right after capsulorrhexis creation with a vertical approach to nucleus splitting, usually into 4 segments (Figure 26-4). Another variation, using an ultrasonic prechopper, easily slides instrumentation into a rock-hard nucleus.

Making the Move to Chop

How can you best move toward chop? First, have all essentials down, including a good intact capsulorrhexis, hydrodissection, hydrodelineation, and good nucleus rotation. Then, rather than entirely removing a whole quadrant, aspirate the apex with ultrasound to impale it with good hold, take a horizontal chopper to the periphery of the fragment, and split it into 2. Repeat for each quadrant until you become completely comfortable using both hands to split a quadrant

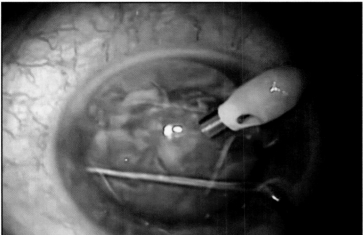

Figure 26-2. To see the difference in chopper placement, this figure shows the horizontal chopper under the anterior capsule and the iris and around the equator of the nucleus. The chopping action will be a horizontal movement toward the phaco tip.

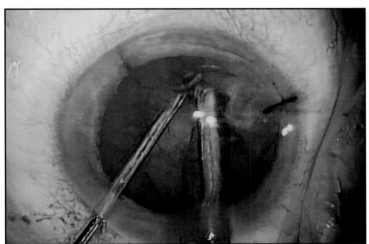

Figure 26-3. Shows the placement of a vertical chopper. Note that it is vertically insinuated into the nucleus with full visualization near the phaco tip. The chopping action is by moving each instrument in opposing directions.

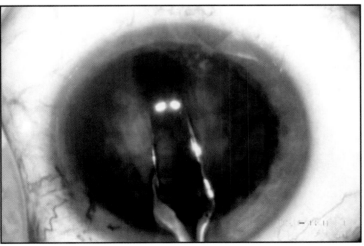

Figure 26-4. A prechopper is in position to split the nucleus in half. This occurs prior to using the phaco instrumentation and usually is used to split the nucleus into 4 to 6 fragments.

into pieces. The harder the nucleus, the more often you should split it so that you gain a sense of improved efficiency of harder fragment removal.

Then, engage the phacoemulsification tip in the trough in the middle of the heminucleus. On the opposite side, place a horizontal chopper and split this heminucleus in two. Experiment by impaling the nucleus using a vertical chopper near the tip to enter down into the nuclear fragment, and split the heminucleus in two. If successful, rotate the remaining nucleus 180 degrees and repeat. If you succeed, you are using the popular stop-and-chop approach. Do not move forward until you are comfortable with these outlined steps.

When you master stop-and-chop and desire to master full chop, it is easiest to start with vertical chop. First, impale the nucleus with the phacoemulsification tip. Make sure the sleeve is pulled back so at least 1.5 mm of the tip is exposed, which aids in maintaining good hold on the nucleus. Vacuum levels of 250 mm Hg or higher are helpful. Place the vertical chopper just in front and slightly to the side of the tip, making sure of a good hold with aspiration. Sink the chopper all the way to the extension end (see Figure 26-3), pull the instruments apart, and separate the nucleus in half.

Common problems include not going deeply enough with both instruments and not chopping aggressively enough for complete separation. Alternately, place a horizontal chopper around the nuclear pole, starting on the central nucleus so you do not get above the anterior capsule and tear zonules. Bring the chopper toward the tip. Just before they contact, do a separating motion to split the nucleus in half completely (see Figure 26-1). When you have two heminuclei, the approach resembles the stop-and-chop method. This is a straightforward, tried-and-true approach to transitioning to chop.

Experienced surgeons find this approach helpful for all cataract density grades. For beginners, very soft and hard nuclei are difficult; do not start with them. With experience, using chop to segment soft or rock-hard cataracts can improve efficiency and safety. I would not approach rock-hard cataracts another way.

Instruments

Many chopping instruments are available. The Lieberman microfinger (ASICO), popularized by Dr. David Chang, is excellent and safe. Horizontal choppers must be rounded and robust where contact to the capsule is not an issue, as you often move without seeing the instrument under the capsule. Do not worry about segmenting a nucleus, even with a small pupil; this becomes a kinesthetic approach not requiring visualization. Vertical choppers generally are sharp. I think those that almost resemble picks are best reserved for experienced choppers. I like a broader bearing surface that would be safe if it contacted the capsule if you did not apply pressure (for example, the Seibel nucleus chopper [Katena Products Inc]).

Conclusion

With attention to detail, it is not difficult to become adept. In my experience, you will never look back and will find chop is your approach going forward.

References

1. Sorensen T, Chan CC, Bradley M, Braga-Mele R, Olson RJ. A comparison of cataract surgical practices in Canada and the United States. *Can J Ophthalmol.* 2012;47(2):131-139.
2. DeBry P, Olson RJ, Crandall AS. Comparison of energy required for phaco-chop and divide and conquer phaco-emulsification. *J Cataract Refract Surg.* 1998;24(5):689-692.
3. Meyer JJ, Kuo AF, Olson RJ. The risk of capsular breakage from phacoemulsification needle contact with the lens capsule: a laboratory study. *Am J Ophthalmol.* 2010;149(6):882-886.
4. Sorensen T, Chan CC, Bradley M, Braga-Mele R, Olson RJ. Ultrasound-induced corneal incision contracture survey in the United States and Canada. *J Cataract Refract Surg.* 2012;38(2):227-233.
5. Nagahara K. Phaco-Chop. Presented at: ASCRS Annual Meeting, U.S. Intraocular Lens Symposium; April 4-7, 1984; Los Angeles, CA.

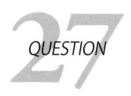

AFTER CHOPPING OR CRACKING A 4+ NUCLEUS, A LEATHERY POSTERIOR PLATE STILL CONNECTS THE FRAGMENTS CENTRALLY. HOW SHOULD I PROCEED?

Roger F. Steinert, MD

The most challenging aspect of phacoemulsification of a 4+ nucleus is the resistance of the posterior nucleus to a clean cleavage of the cracked segments. This is true whether you are performing divide-and-conquer, horizontal chop, or vertical chop.

Understanding the Source of the Problem

To manage the phenomenon, you have to understand its origin. By the time a cataract reaches the 4+ stage, the expansion of the nuclear hardening has incorporated the epinucleus. The posterior epinucleus is no longer a malleable separate cushion layer. Instead, it is firmer and adherent to the endonucleus. When you try to split the endonucleus, the posterior layer has bridging fibers that we have come to call "leathery." Another analogy is the "green-stick fracture" phenomenon that occurs when you try to break a fresh tree branch. The fibers do not break cleanly, but rather flex and keep the two ends of the branch connected.

The net result is that the nuclear fragments you create can be separated, but when trying to engage and remove the fragment with vacuum, it will come only partially and then fall back. The phenomenon of the bridging posterior strands is maximal at the center of the posterior nucleus, which means that the apex of the nuclear fragment not only remains adherent but also cannot be tilted to be engaged by the phaco tip. The result is a stranded posterior plate (Figure 27-1A).

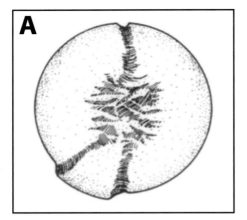

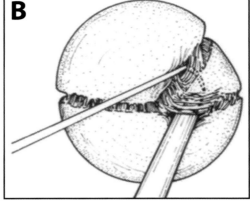

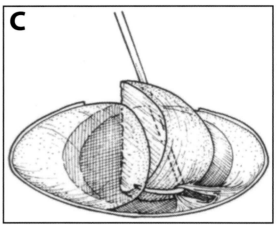

Figure 27-1. (A) Strands of the leathery posterior nucleus are maximal at the apex. (B) The surgeon passes a chopping-type instrument behind the nuclear fragment parallel to the posterior capsule. (C) The chopping instrument snaps the bridging fibers that interfere with delivering and emulsifying the nuclear fragment. (This figure was published in *Cataract Surgery*, Steinert RF, Copyright Elsevier [2002].)[1]

Options

In theory, you might think that flipping the nucleus, so that the posterior portion is now anterior, is the answer. However, even for advocates of nuclear flipping, a 4+ nucleus is the most dangerous type on which to perform this maneuver. The nucleus is very large, and the capsule frequently is more fragile than usual because it is under tension. A very large capsulorrhexis would be needed to flip the nucleus and, even if this were acceptable in regard to later intraocular lens implantation, phaco of a large, hard nucleus in the anterior chamber will result in excessive endothelial damage.

In addressing these 4+ dense nuclei, begin with using trypan blue (VisionBlue; Dutch Ophthalmic) to stain the anterior capsule. This not only aids in performing an optimal capsulorrhexis but also aids in keeping the edge of the anterior capsule visible during the surgery to avoid inadvertent damage to the rhexis and resultant capsular tear. Also, use a dispersive and retentive viscoelastic liberally in the course of the surgery. You will be using a lot of phaco power and have prolonged phaco time, so protecting the endothelium is critical.

I suggest the following specific steps, which have worked for me, to manage the leathery posterior nucleus[1]:

1. Bowl out the center of the nucleus. This spares the endothelium, and the large, firm, peripheral nucleus still provides plenty of material for the phaco tip to grab onto and hold.

2. Use a chopping or finger-type instrument to break the leathery fibers. Although I prefer the hook shape of my claw-shaped chopper (Steinert II Claw Chopper; Rhein Medical), there are many suitable choppers or nuclear-manipulating instruments. The maneuver is to rotate the instrument so that it is parallel to the posterior capsule. While the nuclear fragment is held by vacuum of the phaco tip and drawn partially toward the center, pass the instrument posteriorly under the fragment, from the periphery toward the center, snapping the posterior strands (Figures 27-1B and 27-1C).

3. As soon as you have any area with a visible red reflex, use this space to inject a dispersive viscoelastic (Endocoat; Abbott Medical Optics Inc; or Viscoat; Alcon Laboratories) behind the nucleus. This serves three purposes. First, it creates an artificial epinucleus to protect the posterior capsule. Second, it elevates the nucleus a little, making it easier to pass the instrument posterior to the nuclear fragments to snap the fiber strands. Third, it will stabilize the nuclear fragments, making it easier to position them optimally, avoiding tumbling. Do not forget to add some more viscoelastic anteriorly to protect the endothelium.

Reference

1. Steinert RF. The dense cataract. In: Steinert RF, ed. *Cataract Surgery.* 3rd ed. London, England: Elsevier; 2010.

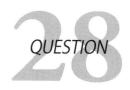

HOW AND WHEN SHOULD I CHANGE MY PHACO AND FLUIDICS SETTINGS IN THE FOLLOWING SITUATIONS: INTRAOPERATIVE FLOPPY IRIS SYNDROME, SHALLOW CHAMBER, HIGH AXIAL LENGTH, AND POSTVITRECTOMY?

Barry Seibel, MD

Phacodynamics involve optimization of machine parameters, as well as microsurgical maneuvers, to facilitate the most effective, efficient, and safest surgery possible for any given clinical situation. Sufficient bottle height maintains anterior chamber pressurization, depth, and stability, whereas excess bottle height can distort iris, zonular, and capsular anatomy, with posterior displacement and excessive anterior chamber depth. Similarly, appropriate aspiration flow rate will facilitate efficient followability of nuclear fragments, while avoiding the excess turbulence that would result from excessive flow rate. Another phacodynamic parameter—vacuum—needs to be adjusted to provide adequate grip of engaged material, but not so excessive that aspiration is produced by the vacuum alone, without the additional modulation of ultrasound energy.

Modifying Actions in Response to Variables

Although certain baseline settings might be effective in a significant percentage of patients (ie, normal anatomy), pertinent modulations must be made, as different clinical factors due to anatomic variations affect the clinical efficacy and safety of a given machine parameter. An example would be the diminished pupil dilation and reduced iris rigidity in intraoperative floppy iris syndrome (IFIS).[1] In this setting, the flaccid iris undulates irregularly out of the iris plane with anterior chamber currents that would otherwise be satisfactory with a normal iris. Furthermore, this unstable iris is in closer proximity to the phaco tip's aspiration port because of the often-inadequate dilation in IFIS. This combination of factors makes it more likely for iris to be aspirated into the phaco tip, causing tissue damage due to vacuum alone, plus possible ultrasound damage. Phacodynamic countermeasures in this setting would include reducing flow and vacuum (Table 28-1). A reduced flow rate will slow the anterior chamber currents and reduce turbulence that causes excessive mobility of the floppy iris. Reduced vacuum will decrease the likelihood

Table 28-1

Phacodynamic Countermeasure Parameters in Response to Intraoperative Variables During Cataract Removal

Clinical Setting	Aspiration Rate	Bottle Height	Vacuum
IFIS	12 to 15 cc/min	40 to 80 cm	0 to 270 mm Hg
Shallow anterior chamber	12 to 15 cc/min	95 to 110 cm	0 to 270 mm Hg
Postvitrectomy	15 cc/min	80 to 95 cm	0 to 200 mm Hg

Abbreviation: IFIS, intraoperative floppy iris syndrome.

of tissue damage in the case of inadvertent iris aspiration. However, reducing these parameters also will decrease the efficiency and efficacy of cataract removal, especially in denser cataracts. A better option in these cases is to maintain appropriate machine parameters for the cataract density, and to enlarge and stabilize the pupil mechanically with iris retractors or a Malyugin Ring (MicroSurgical Technology).

A shallow anterior chamber also presents challenges that can be mitigated with proper machine parameter modulations. The problem lies in the proximity of both the iris and corneal endothelium to the phaco tip, which in a normal-depth anterior chamber would have adequate room. The proximity of the tip can cause potential tissue damage due to ultrasonic energy, even without direct contact,[2] particularly with regard to the corneal endothelium due to turbulent shear force from fluidic currents immediately adjacent to the irrigation and aspiration ports.

As in IFIS cases, the pupil's closer proximity to the phaco tip also increases the risk of incarceration and tissue damage in proportion to the level of vacuum. Reduced flow rate will decrease turbulent currents and shear force in the anterior chamber, and decreased ultrasound energy will reduce the risk of corneal endothelial damage (Table 28-1). Reduced vacuum, as with IFIS cases, will reduce potential iris damage if inadvertently incarcerated. However, also as in IFIS cases, these reduced parameters will reduce the efficiency and efficacy of phacoemulsification, especially in denser nuclei. Vacuum, flow, and ultrasound will not need to be reduced as much, to the extent that the anterior chamber can be deepened. This can be accomplished by increasing the bottle height to increase anterior chamber pressure, after first palpating the globe to insure normal tension and rule out an aqueous misdirection syndrome or choroidal effusion. Anterior chamber depth also can be enhanced by an ophthalmic viscosurgical device, the Ultimate Soft-Shell Technique[3] created by Steve Arshinoff, MD, with a relatively small inner cohesive core, to allow fluid turnover for ultrasonic safety and efficiency, and a relatively large dispersive peripheral shell to help maintain anterior chamber depth.

Postvitrectomy eyes share characteristics of eyes with long axial lengths with regard to phaco surgery, in that the anterior chamber is often excessively deep. In both cases, the etiology can be found in weakened zonules that are typically diffuse in long axial lengths and often focal in postvitrectomy eyes. In addition to a very deep anterior chamber, vitrectomized eyes also display excessively rapid fluctuation in anterior chamber depth due to lack of the cushioning effect of the more viscous vitreous, as compared with a homogeneously aqueous environment throughout

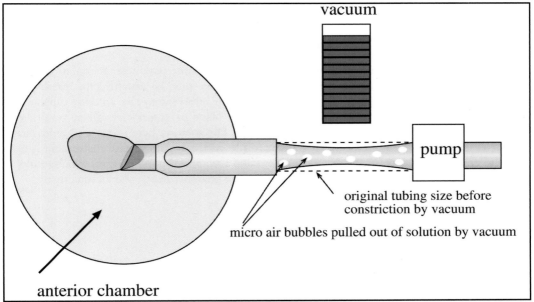

Figure 28-1. When the aspiration tip is occluded, vacuum will build in the tubing. (Reprinted with permission from Seibel BS. *Phacodynamics: Mastering the Tools and Techniques of Phacoemulsification Surgery, Fourth Edition.* Thorofare, NJ: SLACK Incorporated; 2005.)

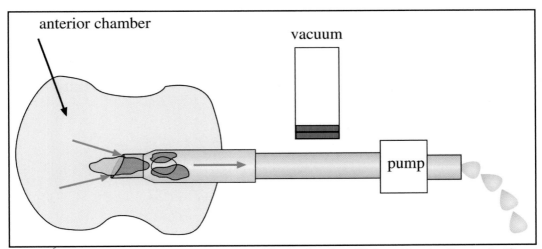

Figure 28-2. When occlusion is broken, a surge of fluid will rush to fill the tubing, leading to significant anterior chamber destabilization. (Reprinted with permission from Seibel BS. *Phacodynamics: Mastering the Tools and Techniques of Phacoemulsification Surgery, Fourth Edition.* Thorofare, NJ: SLACK Incorporated; 2005.)

the eye. Lowering infusion bottle height will reduce anterior chamber pressure and consequently anterior chamber depth in these cases (see Table 28-1). Reducing the aspiration outflow rate will reduce the amplitude of change in anterior chamber depth when occlusion occurs and intraocular pressure changes from hydrodynamic (when outflow is occurring) to hydrostatic (when the aspiration port becomes fully occluded). In these eyes, there is also excessive capsule and iris movement during any postocclusion surges (Figures 28-1 and 28-2). Lowering the vacuum parameter will reduce the amplitude of such surges, as will the use of more restrictive aspiration line tubing, available from most manufacturers, or more restrictive, smaller-bore, phaco needles. These surge-reduction maneuvers are also helpful for the previously discussed conditions of IFIS, as well as shallow anterior chambers.

Managing fluidic challenges does not always involve machine parameter modulations. With high axial length and vitrectomized eyes, the surgeon also must be watchful for iridocapsular block, whereby the overly mobile pupil margin becomes adherent to the anterior capsule and prevents equilibration of pressure posterior to the iris plane or anterior chamber, resulting in significant excess deepening of the anterior chamber. The solution here is not a phacodynamic parameter change but rather a mechanical maneuver in which a blunt second instrument is used gently to create a gap between the capsule and lens and the applied pupil margin, which results in an immediate reestablishment of a more normal anterior chamber depth and architecture.

Conclusion

Intraoperative floppy iris syndrome, shallow anterior chamber, and postvitrectomized eyes represent special circumstances with respect to phacodynamics. Alteration in fluidics settings can greatly lower the risk of intraoperative complications such as iris damage, capsular rupture, and corneal damage.

References

1. Chang DF, Campbell JR. Intraoperative floppy iris syndrome associated with tamsulosin. *J Cataract Refract Surg.* 2005;31(4):664-673.
2. Fishkind WJ. *Pop Goes the Microbubbles*. ESCRS Film Festival Grand Prize Winner, 1998. American Society of Cataract Refractive Surgery.
3. Arshinoff SA. Dispersive-cohesive viscoelastic soft shell technique. *J Cataract Refract Surg.* 1999;25(2):167-173.

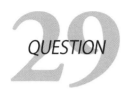

How Do I Recognize and React to a Posterior Capsular Rupture?

Rosa Braga-Mele, MD, MEd, FRCSC and
Theodore J. Christakis, MD

The ophthalmologist that never experiences a posterior capsular rupture is the one that does not operate. However, with preoperative risk stratification, early recognition, and careful management, the frequency and negative implications of this complication can be minimized.

Identify Patients at Higher Risk

An important first step is to identify patients who are at higher risk for rupture. Clearly, an elderly patient with a brunescent cataract, pseudoexfoliation, and a small pupil requires additional care. Patients with previous capsular compromise are also at high risk. Causes of capsular rupture include posterior polar cataract, previous vitrectomy, or a history of intravitreal injections. Finally, one also should recognize risk factors such as male gender, diabetic retinopathy, glaucoma, myopia, and alpha-blocker use, as patients with these risk factors also have an increased chance of capsular tear.[1]

Stabilizing the Chamber Following a Capsular Tear

Posterior capsular compromise can occur even with meticulous surgical technique. The key is to recognize a capsular tear early to minimize any further harm. The earliest signs can be subtle and may manifest as a change in red reflex or a particularly clear area of capsule. You may notice mydriasis or miosis of the pupil or a sudden deepening of the anterior chamber. At this point, the nuclear segments may display poor followability or may begin to sink. If the hyaloid face has been disrupted, the phaco tip may engage vitreous and become occluded.

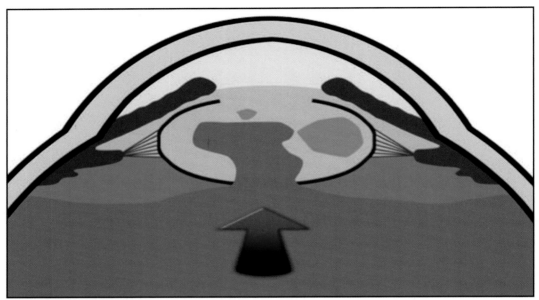

Figure 29-1. Withdrawing irrigation creates a pressure differential between the posterior and anterior segments, which pushes vitreous and intraocular structures forward (arrow) and causes flattening of the anterior chamber.

If this happens, do not panic. Although one's first reaction may be to withdraw the instruments, this would lead to decompression of the anterior chamber, causing extension of the capsular tear and further enabling the vitreous to prolapse forward (Figure 29-1). Instead, maintain the phaco needle's position and continue to irrigate without aspiration. Next, inject a dispersive viscoelastic through the side port in the area of capsular compromise. In addition to stabilizing the anterior chamber, this helps to push back any vitreous and maintains the integrity of the anterior hyaloid face. Only now can the phaco tip be removed from the eye.

Removal of the Nucleus

After the chamber is stabilized, take a moment to examine the capsular rent. If the anterior hyaloid face is intact and the rent is not large or peripheral, one way of stabilizing the remaining capsule is to perform a posterior continuous curvilinear capsulorrhexis.[2] Using capsulorrhexis forceps, try to make the rhexis as small as possible, as it has the tendency to run equatorially. Subsequent removal of nucleus should be done carefully, using either a dispersive viscoelastic bed or a surgical glide for protection. The fluidic settings should be adjusted to account for the compromised chamber. Decrease the bottle height to 30 cm, lower aspiration flow to 20 mL per minute, and lower the maximum vacuum 100 to 150 mm Hg, to minimize any vitreous pulling or anterior chamber bounce.

If there are large fragments of nucleus remaining, they should be phacoemulsified in the anterior chamber. Use dispersive viscoelastic to maintain the chamber and keep vitreous away from the phaco needle (Figure 29-2). If the situation appears precarious, consider conversion to a small-incision extracapsular technique.

If there is vitreous loss, a thorough clean up is required. We will focus on an anterior approach to vitreous loss, as pars plana vitrectomy is discussed in Chapter 33. In both approaches, it is critical

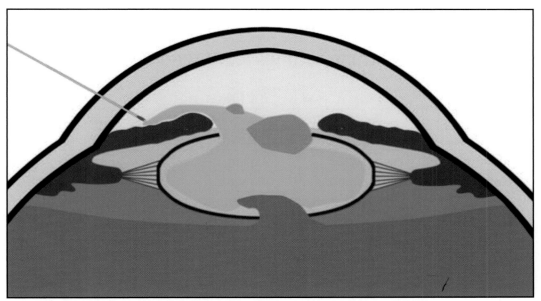

Figure 29-2. Viscoelastic supports nuclear fragments and prevents vitreous prolapse.

to separate irrigation and aspiration, and to remove the sleeve from the vitrectomy probe. When using a bimanual technique, 2 new limbal stab incisions should be created and the main incision closed to prevent vitreous prolapse. Use "I Cut A" (Table 29-1) with a high cut rate (>800 cuts/ min), to minimize vitreous traction, and an elevated bottle height with minimal aspiration (24 cc/ min; 200 mm Hg), to maintain the anterior chamber. Carefully perform an anterior vitrectomy by moving the vitrector slowly over the area of the rent, and remember to sweep the anterior chamber and the main incision. To remove the remaining cortex, switch to "I A Cut," where the aspiration flow rate can be a bit higher. Only activate the cutter if vitreous becomes entangled in the tip. Beware of the tendency to pull vitreous anteriorly toward the wound, which will both increase the amount of vitreous loss, as well as cause retinal traction. Ensure that you sweep the main wound and cut when extracting the instrument from the eye. Also, when trying to cut vitreous from behind the iris, be especially careful not to damage the anterior capsular edge. I use intracameral triamcinolone 10 mg/mL to aid in the visualization of errant strands.[3] However, this often needs to be repeated, as triamcinolone stains only the surface of the vitreous. Although challenging, one must be thorough in removing all vitreous from the anterior chamber.

Intraocular Lens Placement

Intraocular lens (IOL) placement will depend on the stability of the remaining capsule. Sometimes in-the-bag placement is possible if the tear is small and controlled with a posterior continuous curvilinear capsulorrhexis. If not, and the anterior capsule is intact, placing a 3-piece lens in the sulcus and capturing the optic through the rhexis helps to maintain centration.[4] A single-piece IOL should never be placed in the sulcus because of the risk of decentration, uveitis, and hemorrhage. If there appears to be poor capsular support, suturing the haptic to the iris or sclera may help to stabilize and center the lens. Finally, an anterior chamber IOL is a reasonable option when capsular instability precludes posterior chamber placement, particularly if the patient is elderly.

Table 29-1
Selecting Machine Settings for Anterior Vitrectomy

Setting	*I Cut A*	*I A Cut*
Purpose	Remove vitreous	Remove cortical and epinuclear material
Foot-Position 1	Irrigation	Irrigation
Foot-Position 2	Vitrector	Aspiration
Foot-position 3	Aspiration	Vitrector
Cut rate	>800 cut/min	>800 cut/min
Bottle height	90 cm	100 to 110 cm
Aspiration flow rate	24 cc/min	30 cc/min
Vacuum	200 mm Hg	350 mm Hg

Abbreviations: I Cut A, irrigation cut aspiration; I A Cut, irrigation aspiration cut.

At the end of the procedure, I use intracameral Miochol E (acetylcholine chloride) to constrict the pupil and ensure it is round. Sweep all incisions externally with a Weck-Cel sponge (Beaver Visitec) to ensure there are no vitreous stands attached to the wound. After all vitreous traction has been relieved, close every incision site with 10-0 nylon suture to ensure full integrity of the eye. Postoperative eye drops are especially important to help minimize infection, inflammation, intraocular pressure spikes, and cystoid macular edema, as patients with capsular rupture are at higher risk for these complications.

References

1. Narendran N, Jaycock P, Johnston RL, et al. The Cataract National Dataset electronic multicentre audit of 55,567 operations: risk stratification for posterior capsule rupture and vitreous loss. *Eye (Lond)*. 2009;23(1):31-37.
2. Gimbel HV. Posterior capsule tears using phacoemulsification: causes, prevention and management (PCCC). *Eur J Implant Refract Surg*. 1990;2:63-69.
3. Burk SE, Da Mata AP, Snyder ME, et al. Visualizing vitreous using Kenalog suspension. *J Cataract Refract Surg*. 2003;29(4):645-651.
4. Gimbel HV, Debroff BM. Intraocular lens optic capture. *J Cataract Refract Surg*. 2004;30(1):200-206.

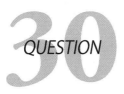

THE ANTERIOR CAPSULE HAS A RADIAL TEAR. HOW DO I PROCEED WITH PHACO AND INTRAOCULAR LENS IMPLANTATION?

Christina S. Moon, MD and
Sonia H. Yoo, MD

A radial tear in the anterior capsule can occur during multiple steps of cataract surgery. Prevention of a radial tear starts by optimizing visualization of the capsule and the surgeon's control over it. In cases of white, brunescent, or dense cortical cataracts, where one can expect it to be harder to see the capsule, the use of trypan blue (VisionBlue; Dutch Ophthalmic) should be considered.

Causes Contributing to Radial Tears

A tear can develop early in the course of surgery, such as during paracentesis construction, viscoelastic insertion, or wound construction, when instruments can nick the capsule and cause an anterior tear in thin capsules. In this situation, and throughout the capsulorrhexis, it is important to ensure sufficient fill of viscoelastic to flatten the surface of the lens and prevent further extension of the tear to the anterior zonules.

In cases where a radial tear is more likely, as with intumescent cataracts, the following may be helpful: (1) use a high molecular weight viscoelastic to flatten the anterior capsule, (2) start the capsulorrhexis with a small diameter, and (3) aspirate the cortex to decompress the capsular bag.

Rescuing the Tear

If a radial tear does develop, it is important to assess how far the tear has extended. If the tear has radialized underneath the iris, the pupil can be pushed back with a second instrument or viscoelastic for better visualization.

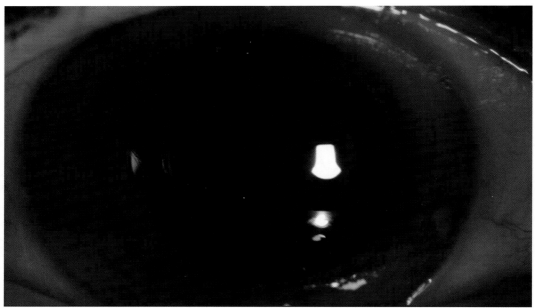

Figure 30-1. Reverse optic capture. (Reprinted with permission from Carol Karp, MD.)

The tear can be rescued using several techniques. Little et al[1] described a technique in which the capsular flap is unfolded flat and pulled backward from the intended direction of the tear to redirect the capsule more centrally. This technique is discussed in Chapter 23. Generous and frequent instillation of viscoelastic should be used during the surgery to keep the anterior capsule flat.

When the tear has gone out to the peripheral zonules and cannot be rescued, there are several options. The surgeon can make a relaxing incision with scissors at the flap edge, continuing in the same direction, or restart the rhexis from the other direction. A traditional can-opener technique also can be used to complete the capsulorrhexis. After completion of the capsulorrhexis, one can perform multiple, gentle hydrodissections away from the area of the rent, to minimize posteriorization of the tear.

After hydrodissection, chopping in the bag with lowered fluidic parameters minimizes the stress on the zonules and the chance that the tear will extend to the posterior capsule. Avoid excessive turning of the lens in the bag during nuclear removal to avoid extension of the tear.

During cortex removal, start with removal of the cortex away from the area of the tear, ending with cortex removal near the area of the tear with dry dissection and generous use of viscoelastic to avoid grasping the tear.

In one retrospective study,[2] intraocular lens (IOL) implantation was the most common step in which an anterior capsule tear extended posteriorly. In cases where the anterior capsule tear has not extended to the posterior capsule, care should be taken to avoid excessive rotation of the lens when it is unfolded, thus minimizing further extension of the tear. We recommend insertion of a 1-piece acrylic IOL, taking care to orient the haptics away from the area of the tear before the lens unfolds in the capsular bag.

In cases where the anterior capsular tear has extended to the posterior capsule, we recommend implanting a 3-piece sulcus lens, with its haptics oriented away from the rent, and reverse optic capture of the bag, if possible, to prevent rotation into the area of the tear or dislocation of the lens over time (Figure 30-1). Haptics should always be placed away from the area of the tear, and care should be taken to avoid excessive turning of the lens in the bag after it has unfolded. This will help minimize further extension of the tear or migration of the haptics through the tear and onto the vitreous face.

References

1. Little BC, Smith JH, Packer M. Little capsulorhexis tear-out rescue. *J Cataract Refract Surg.* 2006;32(9):1420-1422.
2. Marques FF, Marques DMV, Osher RH, Osher JM. Fate of anterior capsule tears during cataract surgery. *J Cataract Refract Surg.* 2006;32(10):1638-1642.

WHEN AND HOW SHOULD I IMPLANT AN INTRAOCULAR LENS IN THE CILIARY SULCUS?

Thomas A. Oetting, MS, MD

An intraocular lens (IOL) often can be securely placed using what remains of a damaged capsule for support.[1] Four typical situations of damaged capsule are: (1) anterior capsular tear without extension, (2) posterior capsular tear with intact anterior capsule, (3) anterior capsular tear extending to a posterior capsular tear, and (4) zonular dehiscence.

Placing the Intraocular Lens in the Sulcus

The most important part of placing an IOL in the sulcus is getting both haptics in the sulcus.[2] The most common problem is to have 1 haptic in the sulcus and the other in the bag, which results in a decentered IOL (Figure 31-1).

One reason it is hard to get both haptics in the sulcus is that the most common area of damage to the capsule is directly across from the wound. This area is vulnerable to radial tears, as ophthalmic viscosurgical devices (OVD) often are running low as the capsulorrhexis passes this point, and the area is vulnerable because the phaco tip and chopper are active in this region. Unfortunately, this same area is where the leading haptic naturally flows during IOL insertion. If the capsule is damaged in this area, then the sulcus is poorly defined, and the leading haptic can end up posterior to the anterior capsule rather than in the sulcus as intended.

When I am faced with capsular damage across from the wound, I often will inject the IOL into the eye and direct the leading haptic anterior to the iris in the anterior chamber to avoid the damaged capsule. I then use Kelman-McPherson forceps to place the trailing haptic into the sulcus, followed by an instrument such as a Sinskey hook to rotate the IOL approximately 90 degrees, so that the haptics are away from the damaged area. I then take the Sinskey hook through a paracentesis, slide it over and hook it onto the leading haptic, and pull the haptic inside the pupil, releasing

Figure 31-1. Decentered IOL. The superior haptics in the sulcus and the inferior haptic is in the bag.

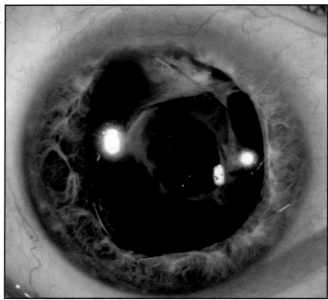

Figure 31-2. Single-piece, acrylic IOL with haptics placed in the sulcus, leading to iris transillumination defects.

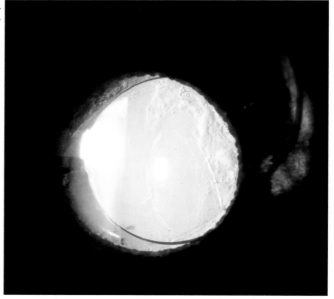

the haptic just under the iris into the sulcus. Defining the sulcus with a viscous OVD (eg, Viscoat; Alcon Laboratories) will greatly ease placement of the haptics.

The second most common problem when placing an IOL in the sulcus is using the wrong IOL design or power. The best IOL for the sulcus has a large optic that is forgiving of mild decentration and permits a better view of the peripheral retina, long haptics with an overall length that will center the IOL (even in large eyes) and smooth, thin haptics to reduce chaffing of the posterior leaf of the iris. Figure 31-2[3] shows a single-piece, acrylic IOL with large, square-edged haptics that was placed in the sulcus, leading to iris transillumination defects and pigmentary glaucoma.

Table 31-1
Preferred Intraocular Lenses for Implantation in the Sulcus

Model	Manu-facturer	Haptic Length	IOL Size	Optic Material	Anterior Edge	Advantages	Disadvantages
AQ2010V	STAAR	13.5	6.3 mm	Silicon	Rounded	Long haptic is great for large eyes; rounded anterior edge	Injects too quickly; material not great if vitrectomy is required
MA50	Alcon	13.0	6.5 mm	Acrylic	Square	Controlled injection; material OK for vitrectomy	Haptic length too small for larger eyes; square edge may rub pupil

Chang et al[3] has proposed the AQ2010V (STAAR Surgical Company) as the preferred sulcus IOL. The AQ2010V is a 3-piece IOL with large silicone optics, a rounded anterior edge, and a long haptic length. I prefer acrylic over silicone IOLs for sulcus implantation because patients with capsular trauma are at increased risk for retinal detachment and the possible use of silicone oil. I often use the MA50 3-piece IOL (Alcon Laboratories) because it has wide haptics, a large yet injectable 6.5-mm optic, and it is acrylic (Table 31-1).

I prefer to inject the IOL into the sulcus rather than use forceps for insertion. Forceps delivery of the IOL requires a larger incision and is not often a familiar technique for the technicians (and surgeons). When injecting the Alcon MA50 IOL, one must be careful not to damage the trailing haptic.[4] Insert the optic into the larger Monarch B (Alcon Laboratories) cartridge as you would a single-piece IOL. Then place the trailing haptic to the side of the knob on the cartridge to protect the haptic from the advancing plunger. While injecting the IOL, make sure the IOL is right side up and the leading haptic is just under the iris and in the sulcus. Leave the trailing haptic outside of the eye until you are sure that the leading haptic is in the sulcus. Finally, place the trailing haptic in the sulcus with forceps or rotate it into the sulcus with a Kuglen hook (Katena Products Inc).

Because an IOL in the sulcus is more anterior than an IOL in the bag, the power of the IOL must be reduced. In a study of 30 sulcus-based IOLs, Maassen et al[5] found that the A-constant should be lowered by approximately 0.80 diopters (D) (Table 31-2). Other studies[6] have had similar results, suggesting that the power of sulcus-based IOLs be decreased by 0.50 D to 1.00 D.

It is very important to eliminate any vitreous in the area of IOL insertion. Vitreous streaming to the wound or to a paracentesis can cause IOL decentration. Careful bimanual anterior vitrectomy, aided with Kenalog (triamcinolone; not approved by the US Food and Drug Administration for this indication), will greatly assist in the long-term stability of the IOL and retina.

There is no need to place a peripheral iridotomy when placing an IOL in the sulcus.

Table 31-2

Power Adjustment for Sulcus Intraocular Lens[6]

	Planned IOL Power (Diopters)	Power Adjustment for Sulcus (Diopters)
IOL in the sulcus	5.00 to 9.00	None
	9.50 to 17.00	Reduce by 0.50
	17.50 to 28.00	Reduce by 1.00
	>28.50	Reduce by 1.50
Haptics in sulcus, and optic in bag	All	None

Abbreviation: IOL, intraocular lens.

Reprinted with permission of Warren E. Hill, MD.

Anterior Capsular Tear With Intact Posterior Capsule

When the anterior capsule has a tear but the posterior capsule remains intact, often an IOL can be placed in the bag. Intraocular lens insertion should be gentle, placing as little stress on the bag as possible. I prefer a single-piece, acrylic IOL in this case because the soft acrylic haptics, oriented 90 degrees away from the tear, create little tension on the bag, thus minimizing the risk of extension of the tear. The single-piece, acrylic IOL is stable in the bag with a radial tear and remains centered (Figure 31-3). The disadvantage to placing this IOL in the bag with an anterior capsular tear is that, should the radial tear advance to the posterior capsule during insertion, the IOL must be removed and exchanged for a 3-piece IOL suitable for the sulcus.

Posterior Capsular Tears With Intact Anterior Capsulotomy

When the posterior capsule is torn and the anterior capsulotomy is intact, you have 2 options for the sulcus and 1 for the bag. One sulcus option is simply to place the IOL in the sulcus. The second is to place the haptics in the sulcus, as described, but then use a Kuglen hook to gently prolapse the optic back into capture by a well-centered anterior capsulotomy (Figure 31-4). This optic capture is very stable and seals off the vitreous from the anterior chamber. With the optic now in the bag, the effective position of the IOL is more posterior, so no adjustment is needed in IOL power (see Table 31-2). The final option applies to stable posterior capsular tears, such as round

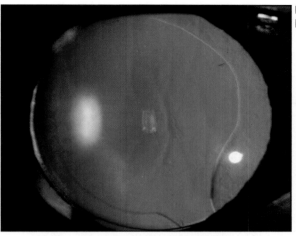

Figure 31-3. Single-piece, acrylic IOL in the bag with a radial tear.

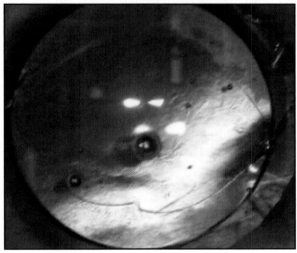

Figure 31-4. IOL with haptics placed in the sulcus and optic in the bag.

holes from a direct phaco needle strike or those tears completed with a posterior capsulorrhexis, which is to place a single-piece, acrylic IOL gently into the bag (Figure 31-5).

Anterior Capsular Tear Extending to Posterior Capsular Tear

When the posterior and anterior capsules are both torn, it is best to seal off the area with Viscoat and to place the IOL in the sulcus as described previously.

Zonular Dehiscence

When the zonules are injured, try placing a capsular tension ring (CTR) with or without a suture. If the area of zonular loss is less than 3 clock-hours, place a conventional CTR. If for some

Figure 31-5. A single-piece, acrylic IOL in the bag with a round hole in the posterior capsule.

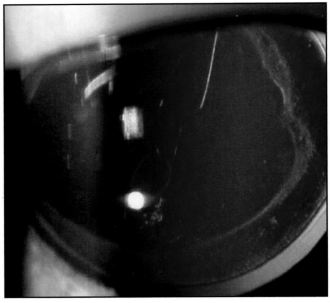

reason a CTR is not available, the IOL will usually remain in position in the sulcus with 3 clock-hours or less of zonular dialysis. If the area of zonular loss is greater than 3 clock-hours, suture a capsular tension segment or a modified Cionni Capsular Tension Ring (FCI Ophthalmics). If not available, be very cautious while placing the IOL in the sulcus with this amount of zonular loss. Try to place the IOL in the sulcus, but have a very low threshold for iris suture fixation.

References

1. Amino K, Yamakawa R. Long-term results of out-of-the-bag intraocular lens implantation. *J Cataract Refract Surg.* 2000;26(2):266-270.
2. Oetting TA. *Cataract Surgery for Greenhorns.* MedRounds Publications, Inc; 2005. http://www.medrounds.org/cataract-surgery-greenhorns. Accessed June 19, 2013.
3. Chang DF, Masket S, Miller KM, et al. Complications of sulcus placement of single-piece acrylic intraocular lenses: recommendations for backup IOL implantation following posterior capsule rupture. *J Cataract Refract Surg.* 2009;35(8):1445-1458.
4. Oetting TA, Beaver HA. Protecting the haptic when a Monarch injector is used. *J Cataract Refract Surg.* 2005;31(2):258-259.
5. Maassen, J, Oetting T, Omphroy L. A constant for sulcus based MA60BM. Paper presented at: University of Iowa Ophthalmology Resident Research Conference; May 19 2006; Iowa City, IA. http://www.medicine.uiowa.edu/uploadedFiles/Departments/Ophthalmology/Content/Research/ResearchDay/2006-resday.pdf. Accessed September 15, 2012.
6. Hill W. Calculating Bag Versus Sulcus IOL Power. http://www.doctor-hill.com/iol-main/bag-sulcus.htm. Accessed June 19, 2013.

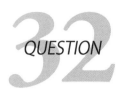

The Capsular Bag Is Unexpectedly Mobile During Phaco. When Should I Implant a Capsular Tension Ring, and Which Size Should I Use?

Iqbal Ike K. Ahmed, MD, FRCSC

Optimal management of weak zonules during phaco is aimed toward maintaining a small-incision, closed system; avoiding vitreous prolapse; preventing further iatrogenic zonular damage; and maintaining the integrity of the capsular bag for in-the-bag posterior chamber intraocular lens (PCIOL) implantation. A variety of capsular support devices are available to help replace the lack of zonular support.

Factors That Determine the Course

The first decision is to determine whether the surgery can continue with a modified phaco technique and adjunctive devices or whether the capsulo-zonular apparatus is compromised so severely that one needs to convert to an intracapsular cataract extraction or extracapsular cataract extraction with or without a pars plana posterior-assisted levitation technique. I reserve this only for the most profound cases of zonular instability or if there is a capsular tear present.[1]

In most cases, phaco can be continued safely with the use of any one or a combination of the following devices: iris or capsular retractors (Figure 32-1), the capsular tension segment (CTS), the capsular tension ring (CTR), or the modified CTR (M-CTR; Figure 32-2). The iris retractor may be placed on a continuous curvilinear capsulorrhexis to support a loose bag, although specially designed retractors for support of the capsular bag provide added support to the capsular equator. Retractor devices provide support of the capsular bag during the operative procedure, while the CTR also provides improved postoperative centration. The CTS and M-CTR are designed for suture fixation to the sclera for more profound zonulopathy.

Iris retractors, which have been designed to open small pupils, or capsular retractors, which are modified for capsular placement, can be of immense use during these weak zonular cases. Every operating room should have these devices available for emergency situations. I find that iris

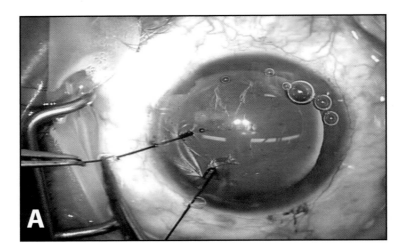

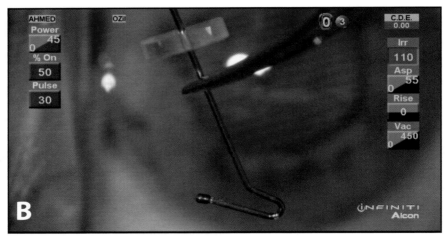

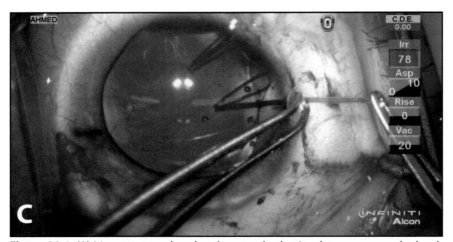

Figure 32-1. (A) Iris retractors placed at the capsulorrhexis edge to support the localized area of zonular weakness. (B) The Mackool capsular retractor (Storz Ophthalmic; Bausch & Lomb Inc). (C) The MST capsular retractor (MicroSurgical Techonology Inc) placed to expand the capsular equator.

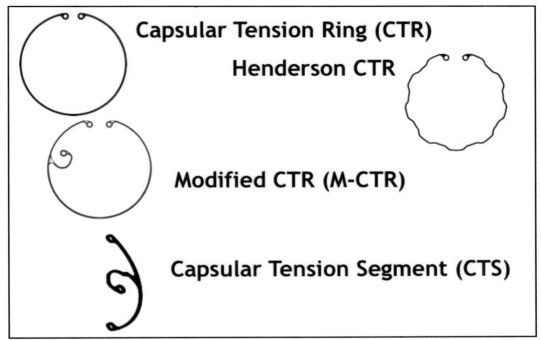

Figure 32-2. Current capsular tension devices.

retractors work reasonably well for this purpose, although specially designed capsular retractors have the right amount of angle and length to support the capsular bag more adequately. Iris retractors are placed on the capsulorrhexis edge to support the anterior capsule, whereas capsular retractors are designed not only to support the capsulorrhexis but also the capsular equator, to center the capsular bag. As many retractors as required are used to support the area(s) of zonular weakness. The retractors act as synthetic zonules that can be placed at any time during the procedure and are particularly useful during completion of the continuous curvilinear capsulorrhexis.

The downsides of these devices include the potential for creating an anterior capsule tear at the point of contact and the possibility of the hooks becoming dislodged or twisted during the procedure. Iris retractors do not expand the capsular equator, which can lead to difficulty during phaco and during cortical stripping, and they may fail to prevent aspiration of a lax capsule. The added support of the capsular retractor to support the capsular equator and place the posterior capsule under tension has additional value here.

The CTR does an excellent job of expanding the capsular equator; however, it can be tricky to insert, as explained later in this chapter. In cases of mild zonular weakness, the CTR alone is sufficient to stabilize the capsular bag; CTRs will not recenter or support the bag in cases of moderate or severe zonular instability. In these more advanced cases, sutured devices should be used.

The CTS can provide the dual benefits of a CTR and capsule retractors because the CTS can be used to expand/fixate the capsule rim in a focal location (as does a capsular retractor) and has a broad internal portion which can expand the capsular equator (as does a CTR). The CTS can be placed easily with the capsular bag at any time during the surgery. To fixate the CTS to the sclera during surgery, an iris retractor is placed through the fixation eyelet.

The selection and the timing of device placement depends primarily on two factors. The first factor is the degree of focal zonulopathy, which is quantified according to the number of clock hours of zonular dialysis or a qualitative assessment of generalized zonular weakness (eg, any

Table 32-1
Zonulopathy Severity Grading

Grade	Zonular Dialysis	Level of Phacodonesis
Minimal	No overt	Minimal
Mild	<4 clock hours	Mild
Moderate	4 to 8 clock hours	Moderate
Severe	>8 clock hours	Severe

phacodonesis?). The second factor is the density of the cataract. I simply grade the zonulopathy as being either minimal, mild, moderate, or severe[1] (Table 32-1).

I use a CTR in all cases with any zonular instability, unless there is an anterior or posterior capsular tear or discontinuity. I use a larger-sized ring (ie, 13 mm) in most cases because this provides greater centrifugal force and ensures adequate overlap of the end terminals.

The main question with CTRs is one of timing, and this may also depend on the lens density. The CTR can be placed anytime after completion of the capsulorrhexis and should be inserted as early as is necessary. Capsular tension ring placement prior to phaco can be accomplished safely in softer- and medium-density cataracts. One key suggestion in placing a CTR before phaco is to perform viscodissection, rather than hydrodissection of the nucleus. Using a cohesive ophthalmic viscosurgical device (OVD) will cleave the cortical–capsular attachments, create space for CTR implantation, and provide enough lubrication to facilitate dialing the CTR into position.

In contrast, with a very dense lens, one needs to weigh the risks and benefits of early versus late insertion because of the potential for the CTR to tear the zonules or the capsule as it is implanted. This is due to the paucity of cortex and epinucleus with dense, bulky cataracts. To delay CTR implantation for as long as possible, iris or capsular retractors, or the CTS, may be used to stabilize the capsular bag during phaco. This also will be discussed later.

Capsular tension ring implantation may be performed either manually or with an injector (Figure 32-3). As it is implanted, the CTR should be directed toward the area of greatest zonular dehiscence to stress the compromised areas as little as possible. A Kuglen (Katena Products Inc) or similar hook can provide countertraction if needed. In cases of advanced zonular weakness, the presence of iris or capsular retractors or the CTS can stabilize the capsular bag against the torque generated as the CTR is inserted.

Phaco Pearls

For eyes with weak zonules, I do not alter my incision to preserve the advantages of a temporal clear corneal approach. If the zonular dialysis is temporal, I place the appropriate device needed to support this area beneath the incision.

In terms of OVD, I prefer a soft-shell technique. A dispersive OVD is used to coat the corneal endothelium and to cover the area of zonular dialysis, while a central cohesive core stabilizes the anterior chamber (AC). In the most severe cases, extra syringes of OVD probably will be neces-

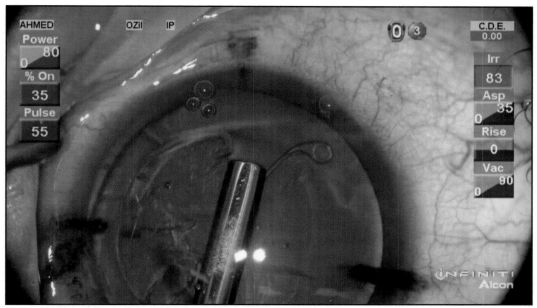

Figure 32-3. Injection of the capsular tension ring.

sary. As nuclear emulsification is nearing completion, placing Healon5 (Abbott Medical Optics Inc) within the capsular bag can prevent the tendency for the capsular bag to collapse inward.

The advantages of a capsulorrhexis are well known but are even more critical in these cases. The capsulorrhexis ideally should be centered, round, and 5 mm in diameter. This size is large enough to facilitate lens removal and to prevent postoperative capsular phimosis and also is sized adequately for placement of iris or capsular retractors or a CTS. This diameter opening also permits continuous edge overlap of the IOL optic.

In cases of moderate to severe zonulopathy, it is important to stabilize the capsular bag with the appropriate device prior to phaco; otherwise, there is increased risk of vitreous prolapse, loss of nuclear fragments, or posterior capsular rupture.

In terms of phaco technique, if the lens is soft, with a healthy cornea and a deep AC, I prefer to flip the nucleus and perform supracapsular phaco. If the circumstances are not appropriate for a phaco flip technique, an endocapsular vertical phaco chop is preferred. It is helpful to lower the fluidics and slow down the procedure in these cases.

It is essential that there be no loss of AC depth during the procedure, particularly during instrument exchange (ie, after phaco or after cortical aspiration). If this should occur, there is a significant risk of vitreous prolapse through or around the weak zonule. Balanced salt solution or an OVD should be injected to prevent loss of AC depth at these times.

If vitreous prolapse is present preoperatively or occurs intraoperatively, a vitrectomy, either bimanual through limbal paracentesis incisions or pars plana with AC infusion, as indicated, should be performed prior to continuation of phaco. However, the vitrectomy should not be initiated until after the capsular bag has been adequately supported and stabilized with the appropriate device. This avoids the potential for posterior dislocation of the nucleus during the vitrectomy.

Device Selection Guidelines

MINIMAL ZONULOPATHY

In these cases, a simple CTR is sufficient, and this may be implanted either early on or at the end of the procedure.[2] Because the zonules are only minimally affected, simply employing a phaco technique that minimizes zonular stress should alone suffice. The indication for the CTR is to provide postoperative IOL centration and support.

MILD ZONULOPATHY

Again, a simple CTR is sufficient. In these cases, it is advantageous to place the CTR as early as possible. I sometimes like to have an iris or capsular retractor placed over the area of dialysis to stabilize this area and to provide countertraction during CTR insertion. The retractors either can be left in until after IOL implantation or removed after CTR implantation. A sutured capsular tension device, such as the CTS or M-CTR, is usually not needed in these cases.

MODERATE ZONULOPATHY

These cases do require a sutured device, either the CTS or M-CTR.[3] I employ iris or capsular retractors while performing the continuous curvilinear capsulorrhexis to re-center the capsular bag and to provide countertraction. Then, place a CTS over the area of zonular dialysis and place an iris retractor within the CTS to support the capsular bag in this quadrant (Figure 32-4). A CTR is then implanted, after which phaco can be performed safely in a well-supported environment.[4]

The CTS can be permanently sutured to the sclera using 9-0 polypropylene or 7-0 Gore-Tex sutures (Figure 32-5). Alternatively, the M-CTR may be used; however, it is difficult to implant this device early in the surgery prior to phaco; thus, one must rely only on iris or capsular retractors until the lens has been evacuated.

SEVERE ZONULOPATHY

The same principles apply as with moderate zonulopathy cases, but typically two CTS devices are required 180 degrees apart. Alternatively, the double-eyelet M-CTR may be used.[5]

Intraocular Lens Selection and Placement

In-the-bag PCIOL placement is by far the ideal location. If the capsular bag has been supported well with a CTR, with or without a sutured device (ie, CTS or M-CTR), this should be a stable environment in the long term. I prefer an acrylic PCIOL, which has less tendency for anterior capsular opacification and capsular contracture that can lead to postoperative decentration.

Although it may be tempting to place a PCIOL in the sulcus in these eyes, I generally avoid this. Unless the zonular deficiency is supported, sulcus IOLs are also at risk for postoperative decentration. One option would be to place a CTR in the bag and a 3-piece PCIOL in the sulcus with optic capture, thereby reducing the risk of capsular contracture, while utilizing the CTR to support the bag, with the haptics of the IOL potentially fibrosing in the ciliary sulcus. Other alternatives, should an in-the-bag PCIOL be deemed risky, include an iris-sutured PCIOL, an iris-claw ARTISAN aphakic IOL (Ophtec BV), or an AC IOL.

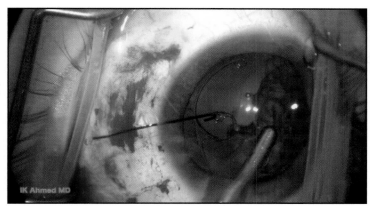

Figure 32-4. CTS placed in area of zonular dialysis with an inverted iris hook through the eyelet for support during surgery.

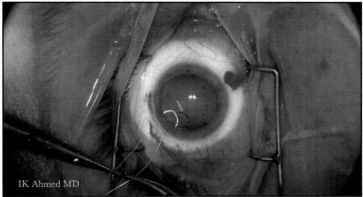

Figure 32-5. CTS fixated to the sclera with Gore-Tex suture.

Postoperative Monitoring

Postoperatively, one must carefully monitor the eye for capsular contracture. If this occurs, neodymium-doped yttrium aluminum garnet (Nd:YAG) laser anterior capsule-relaxing incisions should be performed to release the tension and spread the contracting forces so to avoid IOL decentration.

If postoperative IOL decentration does occur, the lens should be surgically repositioned as soon as possible. The presence of a CTR provides one with the option to pass a polypropylene suture loop under and over the CTR (needle passed through the bag to get under the CTR) so that the CTR becomes fixated to the sclera. Typically 1, 2, or even 3 fixation points may be required.

References

1. Ahmed IIK, Cionni RJ, Kranemann C, Crandall AS. Optimal timing of capsular tension ring implantation: a Miyake-Apple video analysis. *J Cataract Refract Surg.* 2005;31(9):1809-1813.
2. Bayraktar S, Altan T, Küçüksümer Y, Yilmaz OF. Capsular tension ring implantation after capsulorhexis in phaco-emulsification of cataracts associated with pseudoexfoliation syndrome. Intraoperative complications and early postoperative findings. *J Cataract Refract Surg.* 2001;27(10):1620-1628.

3. Cionni RJ, Osher RH. Management of profound zonular dialysis or weakness with a new endocapsular ring designed for scleral fixation. *J Cataract Refract Surg.* 1998;24(10):1299-1306.

4. Hasanee K, Ahmed II. Capsular tension rings: update on endocapsular support devices. *Ophthalmol Clin North Am.* 2006;19(4):507-519.

5. Hasanee K, Butler M, Ahmed II. Capsular tension rings and related devices: current concepts. *Curr Opin Ophthalmol.* 2006;17(1):31-41.

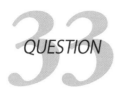

WHEN SHOULD AN ANTERIOR VITRECTOMY BE PERFORMED VIA THE PARS PLANA VERSUS THE LIMBUS?

Louis D. "Skip" Nichamin, MD

Most surgeons would agree that the single most significant complication faced today when performing phaco surgery is rupture of the posterior capsule and vitreous loss. Fortunately, in the setting of small-incision surgery, if the surgeon adheres to certain fundamental principles and uses proper instrumentation and surgical technique, the vast majority of these complicated eyes will enjoy an outcome that differs little from that of an uncomplicated case.[1,2] I believe that adopting a pars plana approach for the vitrectomy is paramount in achieving such results.[3]

Guiding Principles

The guiding principles for this complication include quick recognition of the problem, avoidance of hypotony, and maintenance of a truly closed-chamber environment. This requires the use of watertight incisions. As such, a much lower rate and volume of infusion may be used, thereby reducing intraocular turbulence. To further enhance control of the intraocular environment and to reduce vitreoretinal traction, a separated or bimanual vitrectomy should be utilized. In this way, the location and vector force of the infusion is displaced from the point where one is delicately attempting to remove vitreous. A reasonable approach is to place both instruments through limbal incisions (Figure 33-1).

I would submit, however, that a much more efficient and potentially safer approach in nearly all cases is to perform the vitrectomy through a pars plana incision (Figure 33-2). The only exception to this rule would be in the case of a very limited degree of anterior vitreous prolapse, wherein a limbal approach may be used in concert with a dry (nonirrigating) technique. A pars plana approach better allows the surgeon to "pull down" prolapsed vitreous from the anterior chamber, markedly reducing the amount of vitreous that is removed from the eye. When working from the limbus and bringing vitreous up, it is more difficult to find an end point, and one

Figure 33-1. Bimanual vitrectomy performed through limbal incisions.

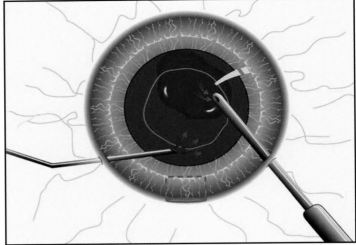

Figure 33-2. Bimanual vitrectomy with vitreous cutter placed through a pars plana incision.

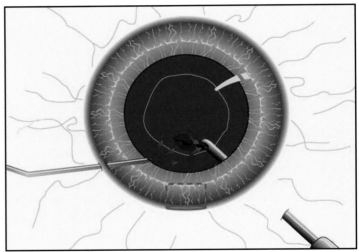

often unintentionally removes a considerable portion of the vitreous body and then must manage a hypotonous eye.

Another significant advantage to working through a pars plana incision is the enhanced access one has to residual lens material. Cortex, epinucleus, and even medium-density nucleus may be removed with the vitrectomy instrument by gradually increasing vacuum and reducing the cutting rate. When addressing vitreous, the highest cut rate is used with the lowest possible vacuum that allows for tissue removal. In this way, a more complete clean up may be achieved, reducing secondary complications such as increased intraocular pressure, inflammation, and cystoid macular edema.

The Pars Plana Approach

It goes without saying that care and effort must be directed toward the learning and acquisition of any new surgical technique, but, in reality, the pars plana approach is quite straightforward.

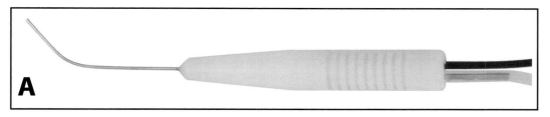

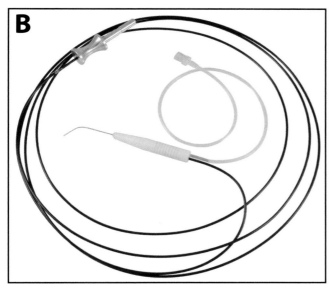

Figure 33-3. (A) Close-up view of the 23-gauge endoilluminated anterior chamber infusion cannula. (B) Cannula with endoillumination and infusion tubing. (Reprinted from *Journal of Cataract and Refractive Surgery*, 38/8, Nichamin LD, Endoilluminated infusion cannula for anterior segment surgery, 1322-1324, 2012, with permission from Elsevier.)

Typically, one first takes down the conjunctiva and applies light cautery at the site of the intended sclerotomy, although some surgeons will incise directly through the conjunctiva. The cardinal meridia should be avoided due to increased vascularity. Given that the posterior capsule is open, infusion may be placed through a limbal paracentesis incision or through a second pars incision. The clock-hour of the vitrectomy incision should be selected to best access remaining lens material.

The pars plana is anatomically located between 3.0 and 4.0 mm posterior to the limbus; so, most commonly, the incision is placed 3.5 mm from the limbus, although an adjustment may be made for unusual axial lengths. Traditionally, wounds were created to accommodate either 19- or 20-gauge instruments. A dedicated disposable microvitreoretinal knife is recommended to create properly sized, and therefore watertight, incisions for both pars plana and limbal incisions. In creating the pars incision, the microvitreoretinal knife blade is held perpendicular to the scleral surface and oriented in a nonradial fashion with regard to the limbus. The blade is directed toward the center of the globe with a simple in-and-out motion. The cardinal meridia are avoided to minimize bleeding. More recently, 23- and 25-gauge instruments have become available, which, in some settings, may allow for sutureless surgery. Insertion using specially designed trocars, however, requires sealing of all open incisions and firming up of the globe. One downside to these smaller and more exquisite instruments is their lack of tensile rigidity and, therefore, the ability to manipulate the position of the globe. Having a dedicated infusion cannula on hand to facilitate a bimanual procedure quickly is also helpful. A new, lighted infusion cannula is now available and is specifically designed to enhance visualization during an anterior vitrectomy (Figure 33-3). In addition, intracameral triamcinolone (Kenalog) may be injected to highlight prolapsed vitreous and can help to reduce postoperative inflammation.

In general, when removing vitreous, the highest possible cut rate is used, along with the lowest possible vacuum setting. One can titrate up with vacuum and down on the cutting rate to remove remaining lens material. Infusion is kept at a minimum—just enough to maintain adequate globe volume.

Care should be taken in both cleaning and closing the pars plana incision. Choices for suture closure would include 9-0 nylon (Ethicon) or 8-0 VICRYL. Prudence would dictate that a pars plana vitrectomy should not be performed for the first time while under duress during a live complication but rather first studied carefully and practiced in a laboratory setting. In this way, a most propitious outcome may be obtained from what remains a daunting complication of cataract surgery.

A final comment should be made in regard to Kelman's novel technique of "posterior assisted levitation," wherein an instrument is placed through a pars plana incision to support or retrieve back into the anterior chamber falling lens material.[4] Although some vitreoretinal experts frown on this maneuver, as it may be associated with limited intraocular visualization, if carefully considered and carried out, it can prevent complete loss of nuclear material into the posterior segment. This technique can be made more efficient and safer by using an ophthalmic viscosurgical device and visco-cannula to elevate the lens material, as described by Chang and Packard.[5]

References

1. Nichamin LD. Prevention pearls and damage control. In: Fishkind, WJ, ed. *Complications in Phacoemulsification*. New York, NY: Thieme Medical Publishers; 2002:260-270.
2. Nichamin LD. Prevention and management of complications. In: Dillman DM, Maloney WF, eds. *Ophthalmology Clinics of North America*. Philadelphia, PA: WB Saunders; 1995:523-538.
3. Nichamin LD. Posterior capsule rupture and vitreous loss: advanced approaches. In: Chang DF, ed. *Phaco Chop: Mastering Techniques, Optimizing Technology and Avoiding Complications*. Thorofare, NJ: SLACK Incorporated; 2004:199-202.
4. Kelman C. New PAL Method May Save Difficult Cataract Cases. *Ophthalmology Times*. 1994;19:51.
5. Chang DF, Packard RB. Posterior assisted levitation for nucleus retrieval using Viscoat after posterior capsule rupture. *J Cataract Refract Surg*. 2003;29(10):1860-1865.

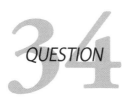

IF I CANNOT PUT THE LENS IN THE BAG OR THE SULCUS, HOW DO I APPROACH SCLERAL FIXATION OF AN INTRAOCULAR LENS?

Richard S. Hoffman, MD

When confronting the clinical scenario of a compromised capsular bag that precludes the use of a sulcus intraocular lens (IOL) or a lens placed in the bag, the surgeon has several options available.

Options

ANTERIOR CHAMBER INTRAOCULAR LENS

The easiest approach is to place an anterior chamber IOL. When properly sized, anterior chamber lenses are tolerated well, and they represent the simplest and least time-consuming method for dealing with aphakia. Unfortunately, instances of chronic discomfort, cystoid macular edema, and corneal endothelial compromise from poorly sized lenses has led to a tendency to avoid their use whenever possible.

POSTERIOR CHAMBER INTRAOCULAR LENS AND IRIS FIXATION

Another popular method for treating aphakia is to insert a posterior chamber IOL and fixate it to the iris. Iris fixation involves much less dissection than scleral fixation, but it has the potential complications of pupil distortion, late hyphema from iris chaffing, and late decentration and dislocation.[1] In addition, when performed in a fully vitrectomized eye, iris fixation can be much more challenging in the presence of an anterior chamber infusion port, thus usually necessitating pars plana infusion and runs the risk of complete IOL dislocation onto the retina during the

Figure 34-1. Limbal grooved incision of 350-μm depth is placed at the 12:00 meridian in this aphakic eye with a previous penetrating keratoplasty.

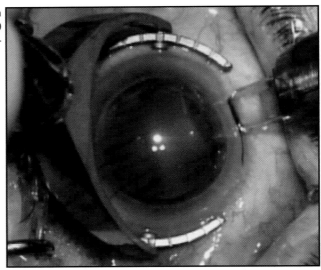

Figure 34-2. Left-sided grooved incision is dissected posteriorly for 3 mm with a metal crescent blade.

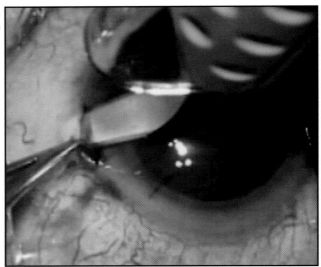

procedure if the iris-captured optic is pulled off of the pupil. Although there are many methods for performing scleral fixation, the following is one technique that allows for placement and fixation of a foldable posterior chamber IOL.

After placement of a dispersive viscoelastic or an anterior chamber infusion port, 2 grooved incisions of 1 to 2 clock-hours in length are placed at the 12:00 and 6:00 meridians. The incisions are created with a diamond or metal step knife at a depth of 350 to 400 μm (Figure 34-1). Each of these grooved incisions is then dissected posteriorly for approximately 3 mm with a metal crescent blade to create 2 corneoscleral pockets 180 degrees apart. Lifting up on the posterior lip of the grooved incision while creating the pockets will facilitate the dissection[2] (Figure 34-2). The dissection is within the plane of the sclera. Marking the lateral extents of the scleral pockets with a gentian violet marker on the conjunctival surface will help to avoid passing sutures through nondissected sclera. If the procedure is performed at the same time as the complicated cataract

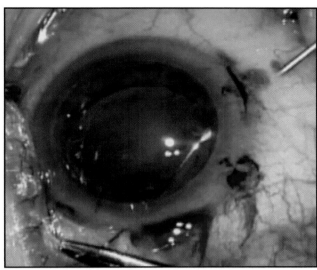

Figure 34-3. A 9-0 Prolene (Ethicon, Inc) long, curved, suture needle is docked into a 27-gauge needle that was passed through the full thickness of the globe, corresponding to the scleral pocket (2 mm posterior to the surgical limbus).

surgery, the temporal clear corneal incision is widened to 3.0 mm for insertion of a foldable IOL and for placement of the 9-0 Prolene fixation sutures.

If present, vitreous should be removed from the anterior chamber with bimanual vitrectomy instrumentation. A 27-gauge needle is then passed through the full thickness of the globe, corresponding to the right-sided scleral pocket, 2 mm posterior to the surgical limbus, and not the conjunctival insertion. The needle passes through the conjunctiva, the roof of the pocket, the floor of the pocket, and through the ciliary sulcus. Take care to angle the needle obliquely to avoid the ciliary processes. One long, curved needle of a double-armed 9-0 Prolene suture is then passed through the temporal clear corneal incision and docked into the 27-gauge needle (Figure 34-3). The curved suture needle usually will lock itself into the straight 27-gauge needle bore so that both can be removed from the globe without internal assistance. The Prolene suture should be 9-0 rather than 10-0 to reduce the risk of late suture breakage and IOL dislocation.[3] The maneuver is then repeated with the needle of the second arm of the double-armed suture, using a new 27-gauge needle passed 1 to 2 mm adjacent to the first pass, 2 mm posterior to the surgical limbus. As the second set of needles are removed from the globe, a loop of Prolene is left outside of the temporal corneal incision to create a cow-hitch knot that will be attached to the leading haptic of the IOL.[4] A small dollop of viscoelastic is placed on the corneal surface to assist in creating the cow-hitch knot. The loop of Prolene suture is then flipped back onto the viscoelastic on the cornea to create the cow-hitch knot (Figure 34-4).

The IOL design for implantation is at the discretion of the surgeon. Unfortunately, there is currently a lack of foldable posterior chamber IOLs with fixation eyelets. For many surgeons, an all poly (methyl methacrylate) (PMMA) IOL with fixation eyelets is the first choice for scleral fixation. This design has the benefit of allowing the suture to pass through the eyelet, avoiding the need for creating knots that fixate the suture to the IOL haptic. Unfortunately, these lenses require larger incisions with greater induced astigmatism, although placing the incision at the temporal location will help to reduce the amount of induced astigmatism. In addition, these eyelet lenses usually need to be special ordered, which may not be feasible in a primary case with a completely compromised capsule. Using a cow-hitch knot allows for the utilization of foldable IOLs, which can be injected through relatively small incisions with a cartridge system.

Treating each end of the foldable IOL's haptics with low-temperature cautery will produce a small enlargement or a frank burr at the end of the haptic that should help prevent suture slippage

Figure 34-4. Enhanced representation of externalized cow-hitch knot preparation.

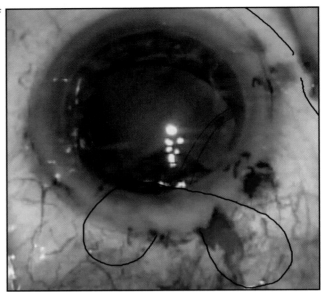

Figure 34-5. Low-temperature, hand-held cautery treatment of the IOL haptic end to help prevent suture slippage.

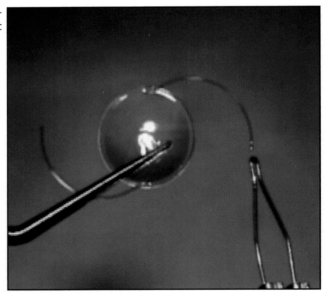

off the haptic. Low-temperature, hand-held cautery (not high temperature), placed close to the tip of the haptic for a very brief second, will create the burr (Figure 34-5). High-temperature cautery or prolonged contact will melt or shrink the haptic, making the IOL unusable. The design of the cow-hitch knot is such that slippage should be avoided if constant traction is placed on the knot and suture as the IOL is inserted.

After preparing the lens, it is inserted in its cartridge injector and extruded enough to allow the leading haptic of the lens to be exposed outside of the cartridge. The leading haptic is then placed through each loop of the cow-hitch knot that was created outside of the temporal incision, and the suture is tightened by pulling on both ends of the Prolene that are exiting from the scleral pocket (Figure 34-6). The haptic is then inserted through the incision, followed by the cartridge, and the

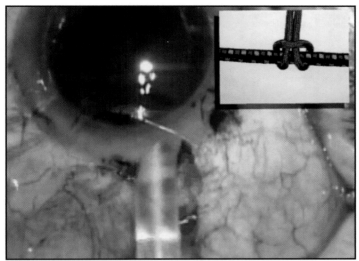

Figure 34-6. Leading haptic of the IOL is placed through the cow-hitch knot while still loaded in the cartridge injector.

IOL is injected into the anterior chamber, leaving the trailing haptic outside of the globe. Gentle traction is placed on the Prolene sutures to help direct the leading haptic toward the ciliary sulcus, taking care to leave the trailing haptic outside of the temporal corneal incision.

The same technique is then repeated for the opposite scleral pocket. A second double-armed Prolene suture is used for the left-sided pocket, and another cow-hitch knot is created and attached to the trailing haptic of the IOL. The trailing haptic is then pulled into the eye by means of traction on the connected Prolene sutures emanating from the corresponding scleral pocket. Starting the fixation process with the right-handed pocket (superior pocket for the left eye, inferior pocket for the right eye) will help to prevent slippage of the suture off of the haptic during IOL insertion. After the IOL has been inserted, both sets of Prolene sutures are tightened to center the IOL.

The needles of the sutures then are removed, and the ends of each set of sutures are retrieved though the opening of the scleral pocket by placing a Sinskey hook (Bausch & Lomb Inc) into the dissected pocket and pulling the ends out though the corneal opening[2] (Figure 34-7). Each set of externalized sutures are then tightened and tied, allowing the knot to slide under the protective roof of the scleral pocket, avoiding the risk of knot erosion through the overlying conjunctiva, with the associated risks of endophthalmitis. No suture closure is necessary for the scleral pockets, and suture closure of the clear corneal incision is at the discretion of the surgeon when all viscoelastic has been removed from the anterior chamber or the anterior chamber infusion is removed from the eye.

Conclusion

Although there are many different approaches for placement of a primary or secondary IOL in the absence of a functional capsular bag, scleral fixation utilizing this technique does offer some inherent benefits. With the use of scleral pockets, suture knots can be created and covered without the need to rotate the knots or the need to perform conjunctival dissection. The use of a cow-hitch knot with this method also allows for the use of a foldable IOL, which should be readily available in most ambulatory surgery centers on the day of surgery. The insertion of a foldable IOL though a 3.0-mm incision, utilizing a cartridge injector, also will lesson the degree of induced astigmatism that might be created with a 6.0- or 7.0-mm all-PMMA lens.

Figure 34-7. Externalization of Prolene suture ends utilizing a Sinskey hook placed into the scleral pocket.

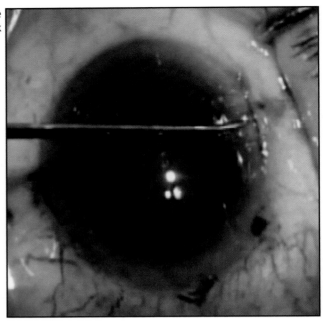

References

1. Kaiura TL, Seedor JA, Koplin RS, Rhee MK, Ritterband DC. Complications arising from iris-fixated posterior chamber intraocular lenses. *J Cataract Refract Surg.* 2005;31(12):2420-2422.
2. Hoffman RS, Fine IH, Packer M. Scleral fixation without conjunctival dissection. *J Cataract Refract Surg.* 2006;32(11):1907-1912.
3. Price MO, Price FW Jr., Werner L, Berlie C, Mamalis N. Late dislocation of scleral-sutured posterior chamber intraocular lenses. *J Cataract Refract Surg.* 2005;31(7):1320-1326.
4. Chen SX, Lee LR, Sii F, Rowley A. Modified cow-hitch suture fixation of transscleral sutured posterior chamber intraocular lenses: long-term safety and efficacy. *J Cataract Refract Surg.* 2008;34(3):452-458.

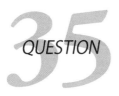

WHEN AND HOW DO I INSERT AN ANTERIOR CHAMBER INTRAOCULAR LENS?

Derek W. DelMonte, MD

Since the first successful intraocular lens (IOL) implantation in the early 1950s, refractive predictability, and thus visual outcomes, has steadily improved. This has made IOL implantation commonplace and has improved the quality of life for countless people throughout the world. Early anterior chamber intraocular lens (AC IOL) designs, including those with 1-piece solid haptics and later rigid closed-loop haptics, soon fell out of favor over concerns of possible corneal compromise and angle damage leading to uveitis, glaucoma, and hemorrhage, known as the UGH syndrome.[1] However, the use of AC IOLs recently has seen resurgence due in large part to technological advances in material and design, leading to increased safety and ease of implantation. In fact, several studies have demonstrated similar outcomes in terms of both efficacy and safety of AC IOLs and sutured posterior chamber intraocular lenses (PC IOL) in patients without adequate posterior lens capsular support.[2,3]

Indications

The current indication for implantation of an AC IOL is lack of sufficient capsular support for implantation of an in-the-bag or sulcus PC IOL. However, many clinical situations lead to the consideration of AC IOL implantation, including secondary IOL implantation in an aphakic patient who has undergone prior cataract extraction; in a patient with subluxed PC IOL, with insufficient remaining capsular support requiring an IOL exchange; or even when the capsular bag is compromised at the time of cataract extraction, resulting in inadequate support for a sulcus lens.

Figure 35-1. Angle-supported IOL design. (Reproduced with permission of Alcon Laboratories.)

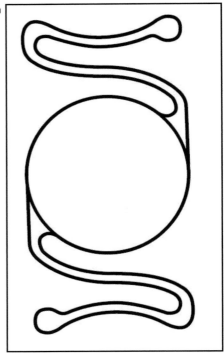

Lens Designs

Prior AC IOLs used closed-loop, angled-supported haptics; however, this design led to many complications, including corneal decompensation and glaucoma.[1] We now have open-loop, angle-supported AC IOLs and iris-supported (iris-claw) AC IOLs, both of which offer improved safety profiles and ease of implantation. Increased optic vaulting and smooth optic edges help to avoid iris chaffing, and flexible concave haptics protect the angle structures to avoid fibrosis and bleeding. Both lens types remain a safe distance from the corneal endothelium and do not require sutures to maintain position.

Angle-supported lenses, such as the MTA-series (MTA2UO to MTA7UO, Alcon Laboratories), have an open-loop, concave, flexible haptic design to minimize contact with the angle, while still maintaining adequate support (Figure 35-1). It is made of poly (methyl methacrylate) (PMMA) and has a 5.5-mm optic and an overall length ranging from 12.0 mm (MTA2UO) to 14.5 mm (MTA7UO) to fit safely in anterior chambers of different diameter.

This lens design is advantageous for its ease of implantation. It does not need any iris support in patients with poor iris tone, lack of iris tissue, or significant iris atrophy. It does, however, require adequate angle support of at least 3 to 4 clock-hours of normal angle in 2 locations 180 degrees apart. Preoperative gonioscopy of the angle is necessary to document the absence of angle recession or peripheral anterior synechia that may prevent safe use of this lens design. In patients without adequate angle structures to support this lens, a scleral-fixated IOL remains the only option.

The ARTISAN Lens (Ophtec BV) is an iris-supported aphakic lens similar in design to the more common phakic Verisyse IOL (Abbott Medical Optics Inc) marketed worldwide for myopia. The aphakic platform is currently available through companionate, special-access programs in the United States. It is made of PMMA, with a length of 8.5 mm, and the central 5-mm optic is supported by 2 unique flexible haptic "claws." As opposed to previous iris clip designs associated with

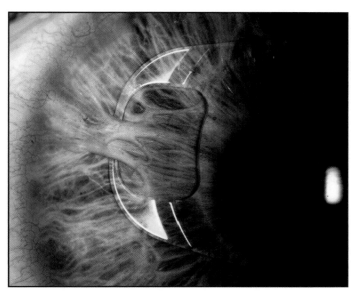

Figure 35-2. Successful placement of an iris-supported aphakic IOL (iris-claw design). (Reprinted with permission of Michael P. Kelly, FOPS Director, Duke Eye Labs, Duke University Hospital.)

iritis, cystoid macular edema, and dislocation, the ARTISAN IOL is fixated to the midperipheral iris and is centered over the pupil (Figure 35-2). In this location, it does not affect mydriasis or iris vasculature, and it does not damage the delicate structures of the angle.

Sizing

Although technically it is easier to implant an AC IOL, appropriate sizing is a concern with angle-supported designs, as angle-to-angle dimensions vary considerably among patients. Incorrectly sized angle-supported lenses can lead to postoperative complications. When sized too large, they can cause pupil ovalization and iritis; when sized too small, they can cause lens instability, endothelial cell loss, and secondary glaucoma. To appropriately size an angle-supported lens, the horizontal white-to-white distance should be measured at the time of surgery. By adding 0.5 to 1.0 mm to this measurement, the surgeon can estimate the diameter of the anterior chamber and select the appropriate sized AC IOL (Table 35-1). Iris-claw (ARTISAN) lenses do not require special sizing, as they do not approach the angle and are supported solely by the midperipheral iris.

Surgical Technique

Prior to placement of either type of AC IOL, several steps must be taken to prepare the eye. Adequate removal of vitreous from the AC and placement of a peripheral iridotomy are most important to avoid future pupillary blockage and acute glaucoma. A laser peripheral iridotomy also may be performed preoperatively—and it should be verified as patent intraoperatively—or postoperatively.

> ## Table 35-1
> # Selecting Anterior Chamber Intraocular Lens Model Based on Size
>
> | White-to-White Measurement (mm) | AC IOL Diameter (mm) | AC IOL Model |
> |---|---|---|
> | 11.0 to 11.5 | 12.0 | MTA2UO |
> | 11.5 to 12.0 | 12.5 | MTA3UO |
> | 12.0 to 12.5 | 13.0 | MTA4UO |
> | 12.5 to 13.0 | 13.5 | MTA5UO |
> | 13.0 to 13.5 | 14.0 | MTA6UO |
> | 13.5 to 14.0 | 14.5 | MTA7UO |
>
> Abbreviation: AC IOL, anterior chamber intraocular lens.

IRIS-SUPPORTED ANTERIOR CHAMBER INTRAOCULAR LENS (ARTISAN)

The ARTISAN iris-claw IOL requires at least 270 degrees of iris tissue, with a pupil size smaller than 6 mm and an anterior chamber depth of at least 3 mm. In some cases, it may be necessary to perform a suture pupilloplasty prior to lens implantation, although the need for this is often known preoperatively. After an adequate anterior vitrectomy is performed, a cohesive viscoelastic is used to maintain the AC and prevent vitreous prolapse. An optional chemical miotic, such as Miochol-E (Novartis Ophthalmics AG), may be used in cases of prior dilation, as during concurrent cataract extraction.

A 5.5- to 6.0-mm incision, which may be made either through a scleral tunnel or corneo-limbal incision, is required to insert the IOL into the eye with nontoothed forceps. When in the AC, the ARTISAN lens is rotated to the desired axis, which is typically horizontal, or in the axis of greatest iris support.

Enclavation of the midperipheral iris into the haptics of the lens is probably the most technically difficult part of the procedure and traditionally has been accomplished using an enclavation needle to sweep the iris up and through the flexible PMMA haptics. Some patients may have a stiff or atrophic iris that makes enclavation difficult, requiring microforceps to help secure the lens to the iris. It is important to remember that, when enclavating iris, 2 contact points are required, one holding the IOL to provide counter resistance and the second lifting the iris into the claw haptics. Because this requires a well-formed AC, I often will suture the large 5.5-mm wound and use 2 paracentesis incisions that help to maintain the AC during this delicate step.

ANGLE-SUPPORTED ANTERIOR CHAMBER INTRAOCULAR LENS

A 6-mm incision is performed through either a scleral tunnel or corneo-limbal incision, and a sheet glide is used to insert the PMMA lens across the AC, which was previously stabilized with a viscoelastic of choice. The trailing haptic then is tucked gently into the subincisional angle, and the whole lens is rotated to the desired location by pulling the supporting haptics centrally and rotating the lens counter clockwise several degrees at a time before releasing the haptic back into the angle. Attention should be given to avoid dragging the haptics in the angle, which will disrupt the delicate anatomy. After the IOL is placed, the wound can be closed and the viscoelastic can be removed with the anterior vitrectomy handpiece.

Postoperative Care

Postoperatively, few changes are required from traditional lens surgery. Careful follow-up is required to evaluate for signs of elevated intraocular pressure, lens instability, or persistent inflammation.

References

1. Apple DJ, Brems RN, Park RB, et al. Anterior chamber lenses. Part I: complications and pathology and a review of designs. *J Cataract Refract Surg.* 1987;13(2):157-174.
2. Donaldson KE, Gorscak JJ, Budenz DL, et al. Anterior chamber and sutured posterior chamber intraocular lenses in eyes with poor capsular support. *J Cataract Refract Surg.* 2005;31(5):903-909.
3. Wagoner MD, Cox TA, Ariyasu RG, J; American Academy of Ophthalmology. Intraocular lens implantation in the absence of capsular support: a report by the American Academy of Ophthalmology. *Ophthalmology.* 2003;110(4):840-859.

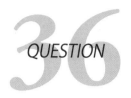

How Do I Proceed if I See a Small Wound Burn With Whitening of Corneal Stroma? How Would I Close a Severe Corneal Burn?

Robert H. Osher, MD

Thermal injuries during phacoemulsification range from a subtle shrinkage of collagen to a dramatic gape of a whitened incision. The former is far more common than appreciated and may appear as a thin, curvilinear lucency in the incisional tunnel, representing contraction of collagen where a focal thermal event has occurred. For example, if the sleeve surrounding the phaco needle is compressed against any part of the tunnel, there may be focal interruption of irrigation and increased friction between the needle and the sleeve. This can cause the temperature to rise high enough to cause the adjacent collagen to contract. Clinically, this is evident as a "shark fin" sign noted as the examiner sweeps a thin slit beam across the incision, observing a subtle curvilinear lucency.[1]

At the other end of the clinical spectrum, complete interruption of either aspiration flow or infusion can cause a rapid and sustained rise in the temperature of the phaco needle. Within seconds, transparency of the adjacent cornea is lost and the surrounding tissue whitens and coagulates, causing the lips of the incision to gape. The incision can no longer self-seal, and frank leakage, with inability to maintain the chamber, occurs. In severe burns, the iris and cornea can be irreparably damaged.[2] What can be done to prevent this serious complication from occurring, and how can the case be salvaged should the surgeon encounter an unexpected thermal injury?

Managing Obstructions

All ultrasound needles create heat by producing friction within the incision. To cool the tip of the vibrating needle, fluid bathes the barrel from the inside (aspiration flow rate) and from the outside (irrigation or infusion). There is also a minor component of fluid leakage around the tip escaping through the incision. The aspiration flow rate is the dominant variable and can be interrupted by obstructing flow with an ophthalmic viscosurgical device (OVD) or by lens material.

The more retentive the OVD, the more likely it is to obstruct the aspiration flow rate, so the surgeon must use enough vacuum to immediately clear a viscoelastic blockage when beginning the emulsification. Moreover, when the aspiration rate is blocked, infusion will cease; there is double trouble at the tip. Because I tend to use highly retentive Healon5 (Abbott Medical Optics Inc), I must embed the ultrasound tip directly into the central anterior cortex bevel down at an initial level of 250 mm Hg, high enough to remove the emulsified lens material without the risk of OVD obstruction. After a divot is created in the lens and there is a safe space for fluid exchange, I reduce the vacuum in accord with the principles of slow-motion phacoemulsification to retain the OVD in the anterior chamber.[3]

The importance of proper incision construction cannot be overemphasized. As surgeons make smaller watertight incisions, which tend to extend more anteriorly into clear cornea, there is a greater risk for compressing the surrounding tubing through which the irrigation passes. Inadvertent "oar locking" or improper pivoting of the handpiece may kink the tubing, interrupting infusion as heat is transferred through the sleeve directly to the cornea. Even a partial obstruction may result in a focal temperature rise within the incision. Moreover, leakage also may be reduced in these tight incisions, so irrigation can occur only during aspiration. If the tip becomes occluded, both irrigation and aspiration are restricted, and the temperature rises. Irrigating choppers also have reduced infusion rates, and the lower-pressure head may not easily move a chamber full of OVD while a sleeveless ultrasound needle is vibrating in a second incision.

During the past several years, manufacturers have added important thermal protective safeguards. All contemporary machines allow the surgeon to modulate ultrasound energy. Because friction is the dominant variable for generating heat, continuous ultrasound is the least safe option. Delivering pulses, or bursts, of ultrasound energy can reduce total energy. Increasing off time by lowering duty cycle is another extremely effective method in reducing heat within the incision. This innovation was introduced by the WHITESTAR technology (Abbott Medical Optics Inc). A dramatic reduction in friction and temperature has been measured with the newest Alcon Laboratories technology of torsional ultrasound. Different tips have been designed to maintain some flow, including the Mackool tip (Alcon Laboratories), which has a rigid outer sleeve, and the Barrett tip (Bausch & Lomb Inc), which has a series of longitudinal grooves that ensure infusion, even if the sleeve is compressed. The ABS tip (Alcon Laboratories) allows fluid to bypass an obstruction until the rising vacuum can clear the occlusion. Audible tones can warn the surgeon when occlusion occurs or when the amount of the fluid in the bottle is low.

Our laboratory studies evaluated the impact of different parameters contributing to incisional temperatures.[4] Power, duty cycle, aspiration rate, viscoelastic, vacuum, and incision size-to-tip ratio have major thermal effects. Pulse frequency, cooling the balanced salt solution, or raising the bottle height had minimal effect. A subsequent study demonstrated a thermoprotective benefit of using a coaxial setup with ultrasleeve to allow a further reduction in incision size to 2.2 mm.[5]

The universal warning sign of thermal injury is the appearance of visible lens particles (lens milk), which represents the stagnant emulsion going nowhere. The surgeon may also notice the lack of cutting activity or lens movement when the tip is obstructed. The surgeon must immediately abort the emulsification by decelerating the foot pedal into irrigation and aspiration or irrigation mode to avoid a rapid temperature rise. Warning beeps or audible tones will alert the surgeon to an interruption of flow, which can be verified by the nurse who quickly confirms the absence of activity in the drip chamber. Although the surgeon may feel a temperature rise in the handpiece itself, the damage occurs in several seconds and has usually occured by this point.

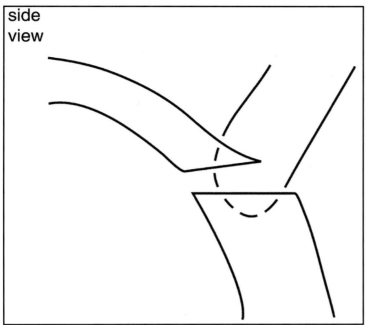

side
view

Figure 36-1. Radial "gape" suture technique. The needle passes through the proximal lip of the incision, then catches a bite of floor before exiting within the gape.

What Do I Do if My Patient Has an Incisional Burn?

If the thermal injury is minimal, you may be able to complete the procedure without much fanfare. Hydration probably will fail to produce a watertight incision, in which case suture closure likely will be necessary. If the injury is more severe and a gape is present, an air bubble or an OVD may be required to prevent chamber collapse while suturing the incision is attempted. Unfortunately, a standard closure is ineffective, because the incision lips are separated as if tissue had been lost. Standard suturing techniques may result in a leaking wound with extreme astigmatism.

The Gape Stitch

We have developed 2 suturing options, a radial and a horizontal "gape stitch," for this purpose. The radial suture begins with the needle entering the proximal lip of the incision, then catching a bite of the floor before exiting without passing through the distal lip[6] (Figure 36-1). This method simply approximates the anterior portion of the incision, permitting a watertight closure.

The horizontal gape stitch is a trapezoidal mattress suture that begins by passing the needle of a 10-0 nylon suture radially through the posterior roof and then exiting within the incisional tunnel[7] (Figure 36-2). The needle is reloaded and passed parallel to the incision through the anterior floor, exiting within the tunnel. The needle is reloaded for a third time, passing a radial bite from within the tunnel up through the posterior roof. The bites through the posterior roof are slightly closer together than the bites through the anterior floor, resulting in a trapezoidal configuration. The sutures are cinched and tied, bringing the anterior floor to the posterior roof and "giving back" tissue for a watertight enclosure.

Figure 36-2. Trapezoidal "gape" suture. (A) First pass: the needle enters radially through the roof, exiting within the incisional bed. (B) Second pass: the needle is reloaded for a tangential pass through the anterior floor of the bed. Both the entry and exit sites are just lateral to the radial meridian so to create trapezoidal configuration. (C) Third pass: the needle is reloaded, entering the tunnel to penetrate and exit through the roof. (D) The free ends of the suture are cinched and tied to form a (E) trapezoidal vertical-mattress suture approximating the posterior roof to the anterior floor.

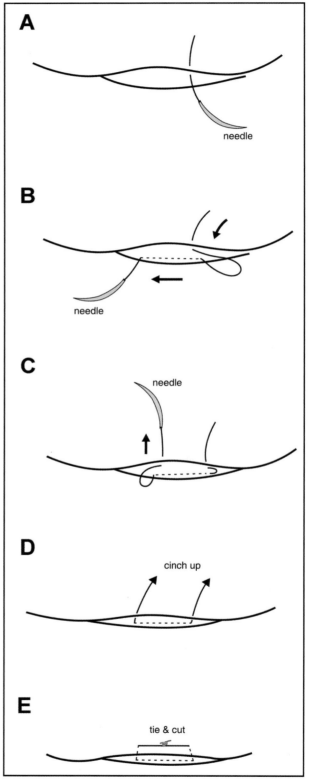

Extreme cases may require a patch graft. However, that discussion is beyond the scope of this chapter.

Conclusion

Thermal injuries are going to occur as a complication of phacoemulsification. However, we can reduce the risk by meticulous surgical technique and the knowledgeable selection of phaco parameters. Remember, if you see lens milk, stop and figure out the problem before resuming the emulsification. Should a burn occur, try to secure the incision with a gape-suturing technique.

Acknowledgment

I would like to thank Scott E. Burk, MD, PhD, and James M. Osher, MS, for their assistance in writing this chapter.

References

1. Osher RH. Shark fin: a new sign of thermal injury. *J Cataract Refract Surg.* 2005;31(3):640-642.
2. Sugar A, Schertzer RM. Clinical course of phacoemulsification wound burns. *J Cataract Refract Surg.* 1999;25(5):688-692.
3. Osher RH, Marques DM, Marques FF, et al. Slow-motion phacoemulsification technique. *Techniques in Ophthalmology.* 2003;1(2):73-79.
4. Osher RH, Injev V. Thermal study of bare tips with various system parameters and incision sizes. *J Cataract Refract Surg.* 2006;32(5):867-872.
5. Osher RH, Injev V. Microcoaxial phacoemulsification: laboratory study. *J Cataract Refract Surg.* 2007;33(3):401-407.
6. Osher RH. Gape stitch. *Video. J Cataract Refract Surg.* 1990;VI(3).
7. Osher RH. Thermal burns. *Video. J Cataract Refract Surg.* 1993;IX(3).

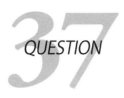
How Should I Manage a Small or Large Descemet's Membrane Detachment That Occurs During Cataract Surgery?

Terry Kim, MD

The incidence of Descemet's membrane (DM) detachments has been cited to be as high as 43%,[1] and cataract surgery has been reported to be a major predisposing factor.[2] Fortunately, the majority of these detachments are small, localized to the wound(s), and clinically insignificant. However, at times, these small detachments can extend during surgery to become moderate- or large-sized detachments that require attention and treatment.

Causes of Descemet's Membrane Detachments

In cataract surgery, DM detachments usually occur at the site of the clear corneal wound or paracentesis incision. By far, the most common cause is a dull blade that causes a focal tear or separation of DM from the stroma (Figure 37-1). The repeated introduction of instruments and devices through these wounds (eg, the phacoemulsification tip, irrigation or aspiration tip, viscoelastic cannula, balanced salt solution [BSS] cannula, intraocular lens [IOL] cartridge, and IOL) can cause these localized tears or detachments to extend and enlarge. In particular, any blunt edge of an instrument or device (eg, the sleeve of the phaco tip, the irrigation or aspiration tips, the tip of the IOL cartridge, and the edge of the IOL) can catch the edge of DM during entry into the clear corneal wound and further strip the membrane (Figure 37-2). Forceful insertion of a viscoelastic or BSS cannula tip or a second instrument (eg, Koch nucleus spatula or Kuglen hook; Katena Products Inc) through the paracentesis incision also can cause DM to tear and detach. The injection of BSS or viscoelastic prior to complete entry of the cannula tip into the anterior chamber also can cause severe DM detachments.

Because these detachments start in the peripheral cornea at the internal incision sites and then extend centrally, they can be difficult to detect and visualize. After wound construction, the surgeon typically is focused on the central aspects of the cornea, anterior chamber, and lens

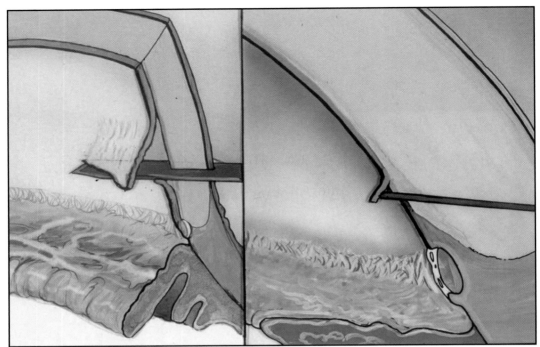

Figure 37-1. This illustration depicts how a dull blade can cause Descemet's membrane to tear or separate from the corneal stroma. (Reprinted with permission from Fishkind W. *Complications in Phacoemulsification: Avoidance, Recognition, and Management.* New York: Thieme Medical Publishers. 2002.)

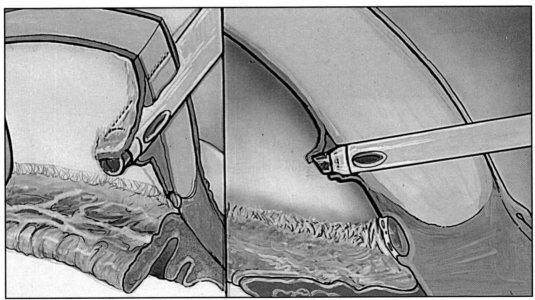

Figure 37-2. This diagram demonstrates how small Descemet's membrane tears, or detachments, can enlarge or extend on insertion of an instrument through the corneal incision. (Reprinted with permission from Fishkind W. *Complications in Phacoemulsification: Avoidance, Recognition, and Management.* New York: Thieme Medical Publishers. 2002.)

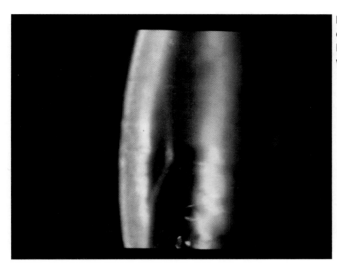

Figure 37-3. Slit-lamp photograph demonstrating a paracentral, localized Descemet's membrane detachment with no evidence of tearing or scrolling.

during the cataract extraction. Furthermore, common conditions, such as arcus senilis and stromal hydration or edema of the corneal wounds, prohibit good visualization of the posterior layers of the peripheral cornea. When these defects in DM are noted intraoperatively, they are recognized incidentally as a torn edge or scroll of Descemet's membrane during instrument or device insertion or, if more extensive, as a frank DM detachment flapping in the anterior chamber during cataract surgery (Figure 37-3).

Prevention

The following routine steps can be taken during cataract surgery to help prevent tears or detachments of DM:

- First, use a sharp blade, whether it is metal or diamond, for all incisions. If any substantial resistance during wound construction is encountered, the blade should be removed, inspected, and preferably replaced with a new blade.

- Avoid forceful insertion of any instrument or device by altering the angle of insertion or enlarging the clear corneal or paracentesis incision.

- Ensure that the cannula tip has passed completely through the cornea into the anterior chamber before initiating injection of viscoelastic or other substances into the anterior chamber so to prevent dissection of DM from the stroma.

As soon as a DM tear or detachment is noted intraoperatively, the following precautions should be taken to avoid further damage to DM, particularly the anterior portion that lies superior to the incision site because of its potential to extend centrally:

- Special attention should be given to posterior corneal abnormalities, particularly Fuchs' endothelial dystrophy. These conditions probably predispose the patient to easier stripping of DM during cataract surgery, due to a compromised endothelial pump.[3]

- Careful visualization of instruments and devices under higher magnification during insertion can help to prevent catching DM.

Figure 37-4. A 20% sulfur hexafluoride gas bubble fills 60% of the anterior chamber to tamponade a large, central Descemet's membrane detachment.

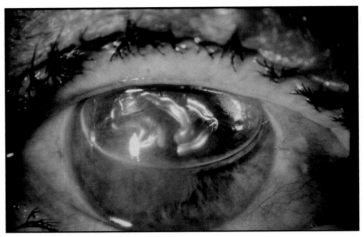

- Because it is more crucial to avoid the anterior portion of DM, placing more posterior pressure on the posterior lip of the incision during instrument or device insertion can help to avoid further stripping of DM centrally.

- Enlarging the incision and lubricating the incision with viscoelastic can ease the entry of instrument or device insertion through a tight wound.

- Using a dispersive (Viscoat; Alcon Laboratories) or adaptive (Healon5; Abbott Medical Optics Inc) viscoelastic can provide a temporary tamponade of the detachment. An alternate incision site is recommended (ie, the paracentesis incision is used for viscoelastic tamponade of DM detachment at the clear corneal incision and vice versa), and extra precaution needs to be taken to ensure that viscoelastic is not injected between DM and the stroma.

Treatment

For small DM detachments noted intraoperatively, no particular treatment is generally necessary. However, moderate- or large-sized detachments may necessitate aborting the cataract procedure and warrant intraoperative treatment with either air or gas tamponade, or perhaps suturing, at the conclusion of the case. The DM tear or scroll may need to be repositioned prior to tamponade treatment and, if so, excessive manipulation and direct contact with DM with any instrument should be avoided to minimize endothelial loss. If the detached DM is too torn, shredded, or scrolled, air or gas injection alone will not suffice. Intracameral air injection lasts a shorter time than gas and should be used for smaller detachments. For more extensive DM detachments, I recommend the injection of a nonexpansive 20% concentration of sulfur hexafluoride gas with approximately 60% to 70% fill of the anterior chamber (Figure 37-4). With either air or gas injection, proper head positioning may be required to ensure that the bubble is positioned correctly against the DM. These patients should be followed closely for intraocular pressure monitoring and DM reattachment, and they should be given cycloplegic medications to avoid pupillary block glaucoma.

Frequently, DM detachments are not noted until slit-lamp examination is performed postoperatively. Clinically, these patients can present with severe corneal edema overlying the DM detachment, which can make the diagnosis difficult. The use of topical glycerin to clear the edema temporarily or imaging modalities (ie, anterior segment optical coherence tomography or

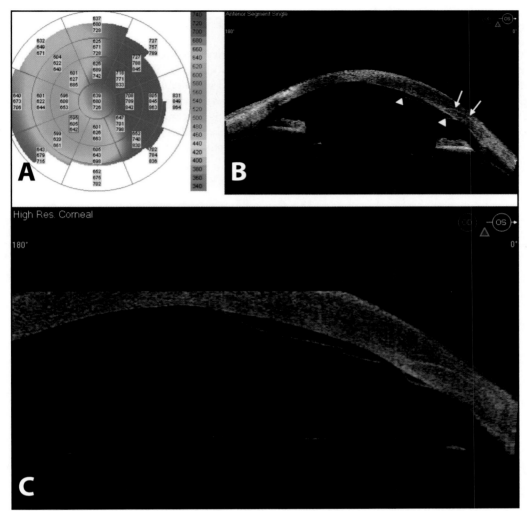

Figure 37-5. Anterior-segment optical coherence tomography of Descemet's membrane detachment after cataract surgery. The orientation of these scans is nasal to temporal going from left to right. The pachymetric map (A) shows sectoral edema temporally, as indicated by the cooler, darker blues. The view of the anterior segment (B) shows the temporal clear corneal wound (arrows) and DM detached from the cornea proper (arrowheads). The bottom image (C) provides a higher resolution view.

ultrasound biomicroscopy) can help to confirm the diagnosis (Figure 37-5). Topical corticosteroid therapy and observation are usually the first steps of treatment, with the hopes of spontaneous DM reattachment. For persistent DM detachments, the same aforementioned techniques utilizing air or gas can be used to reattach DM. Of note, we published a simplified technique[4] for reattaching DM detachments postoperatively using intracameral 20% sulfur hexafluoride gas. It can be performed with minimal instruments in a minor operating room or at the slit-lamp microscope.[4] Finally, various transcorneal suturing techniques may be necessary to address the more severe and refractory DM detachments.[5]

Prognosis

The prognosis for small to moderate DM detachments remains excellent, especially with the more recently described technique of intracameral gas injection. However, permanent corneal decompensation can ensue with severe detachments and will require corneal transplantation. In this scenario, a posterior lamellar approach (ie, Descemet's stripping endothelial keratoplasty) can help minimize incision size, reduce postoperative astigmatism, and hasten visual recovery. In general, the surprising resiliency of the corneal endothelium allows these cells to remain viable, even in the state of DM detachment, so that continued pump function can resume upon successful treatment.

References

1. Monroe WD. Gonioscopy after cataract extraction. *South Med J.* 1971;64(9):1122-1124.
2. Pieramici D, Green WR, Stark WJ. Stripping of Descemet's membrane: a clinicopathologic correlation. *Ophthalmic Surg.* 1994;25(4):226-231.
3. Ti SE, Chee SP, Tan DT, Yang YN, Shuang SL. Descemet membrane detachment after phacoemulsification surgery: risk factors and success of air bubble tamponade. *Cornea.* 2013;32(4):454-459.
4. Kim T, Hasan SA. A new technique for repairing Descemet membrane detachments using intracameral gas injection. *Arch Ophthalmol.* 2002;120(2):181-183.
5. Olson RJ. Corneal problems associated with phacoemulsification. In: Fishkind WJ, ed. *Complications in Phacoemulsification: Recognition, Avoidance, and Management.* New York, NY: Thieme Medical Publishing; 2002.

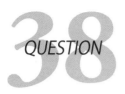
WHAT SHOULD I DO DIFFERENTLY WITH A POSTERIOR POLAR CATARACT?

Robert J. Cionni, MD

It is well known that the posterior polar cataract (Figure 38-1) has a higher risk for posterior capsular rupture, especially if one attempts to perform cataract surgery in a routine manner.[1] Therefore, several routine maneuvers should be altered to decrease the risk of violating the posterior capsule or extending a preexisting posterior capsular opening. Taking these precautions also allows the surgeon to better manage an open posterior capsule.

Precautions

As a general rule, never let the anterior chamber shallow. Properly fashioned, self-sealing incisions, combined with the ample use of viscoelastic agents, will help to maintain a deep chamber throughout the procedure. My preference is for a dispersive ophthalmic viscosurgical device (OVD), such as Viscoat (Alcon Laboratories). It has excellent retention properties in the anterior chamber so that, as aspiration of lenticular debris proceeds, the OVD is not removed all at once, as occurs with more cohesive OVDs.

Make certain that a well-centered capsulotomy is obtained. Ideally, the capsulotomy should be approximately 5.0 to 5.5 mm in diameter. Thereby, if a large posterior capsule opening develops, one can be ensured of a centered and stable posterior chamber intraocular lens (IOL) by placing a 3-piece IOL in the sulcus and capturing the optic posteriorly through the appropriately sized and centered anterior capsulotomy. In these cases, I prefer to utilize the LenSx femtosecond cataract laser (Alcon Laboratories) to assure that the capsulotomy is perfectly sized and centered. However, the lens-chop step is disabled in these cases to avoid any build-up of intralenticular pressure from the gases formed by the laser lens-chop process.

As previously mentioned, one needs to avoid excessive intralenticular pressure from any source. Pressure from within the capsular bag will challenge an already thin and vulnerable central

Figure 38-1. Posterior polar cataract.

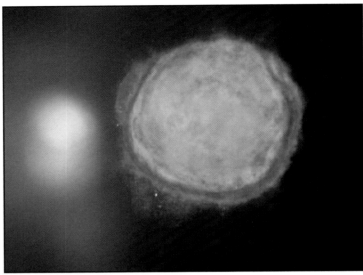

posterior capsule. Hydrodissection represents the most significant source of excessive intralenticular pressure and should be avoided in these cases. Gentle hydrodelineation is felt to be less problematic, but still causes some pressure increase within the capsular bag; therefore, I do not perform either hydrodissection or hydrodelineation in these cases.

Useful Techniques

Without hydrodissection, the lens is not free from the cortex or the peripheral capsule. I fall back on older techniques to remove the nucleus. My technique varies, depending on nuclear density. Fortunately, most of these patients present at a younger age due to the presence of posterior polar and, eventually, posterior subcapsular opacities in the visual axis. In these cases, I bowl out the central nucleus down to, but not including, the posterior polar opacity. With the nucleus debulked, I then can viscodissect the peripheral nuclear and cortical material to move it centrally. By utilizing a dispersive OVD, a barrier moves along the posterior capsule to prevent vitreous prolapse, should there be an opening in the capsule. The peripheral lens material is then removed easily.

In denser cataracts, I bowl out a little less aggressively and then create a very shallow, but wide, groove down to the posterior polar opacity. By placing 2 instruments on the posterior opacity and applying gentle pressure equally toward the capsular bag periphery, the nucleus is divided with very little pressure on the central posterior capsule. A dispersive OVD is injected into the central crevice to lift each half anteriorly and to protect the central capsule from damage or from vitreous prolapse, should the capsule already be compromised.

I strongly prefer a single-piece, hydrophobic acrylic IOL in these cases, as the haptic forces are gentle enough to reduce the risk that haptic-induced expansile forces will test the strength of the central posterior capsule. If an opening is present, I typically then implant a 3-piece, hydrophobic acrylic IOL into the sulcus and capture the optic posteriorly through the anterior capsule.

Conclusion

By treating each posterior polar cataract as if there is already a posterior capsule violation from the beginning of the surgery to the end, one can obviate serious complications. If an opening is found, careful management (as previously outlined) likely will maintain an intact anterior hyaloid, prevent vitreous prolapse, and allow for in-the-bag IOL implantation. Having the proper instrumentation and staff experienced in these challenges will increase the likelihood of a good outcome.

Reference

1. Osher R, Yu B, Koch D. Posterior polar cataracts: a predisposition to intraoperative posterior capsular rupture. *J Cataract Refract Surg.* 1990;16(2):157-162.

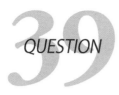

WHAT SHOULD I DO DIFFERENTLY WITH A HYPERMATURE WHITE CATARACT?

Uday Devgan, MD

White cataracts are not all the same, with the principal differentiating factor being the lens nuclear density and the presence of milky fluid within an intumescent capsular bag. A hypermature cataract contains milky-white fluid within the capsular bag. These white intumescent cataracts pose a challenge during capsulorrhexis creation because the intralenticular pressure increases as the lens cortex liquefies.[1]

Managing Pressure

In a routine cataract, the lens material is solid and the pressure within the capsular bag is lower than the pressure in the anterior chamber, making capsulorrhexis creation straightforward. With the white intumescent cataract, the liquefied cortex increases the intracapsular pressure and forces the capsular bag to rip uncontrollably as soon as it is opened. With the capsule stained with trypan blue dye, this uncontrolled radialization of the capsule toward the zonules gives the blue-white-blue appearance of the Argentinian flag (Figure 39-1), which is why this complication is often referred to as the Argentinian flag sign.

AVOIDING ARGENTINIAN FLAG SIGN

The way to avoid development of the Argentinian flag sign and capsular radialization is to keep the anterior chamber pressure higher than the intralenticular pressure during capsulorrhexis creation. Make just one small paracentesis and stain the capsule with trypan blue dye (VisionBlue; Dutch Ophthalmic). Now, fill the anterior chamber with a cohesive viscoelastic until the intraocular pressure is high (40 mm Hg or more). The capsulorrhexis is made only via this small para-

Figure 39-1. Due to high pressure within the capsular bag, the nucleus pushed forward and caused the capsulorrhexis to radialize towards the lens equator, causing the characteristic blue-white-blue appearance, which is often referred to as the Argentinian flag sign.

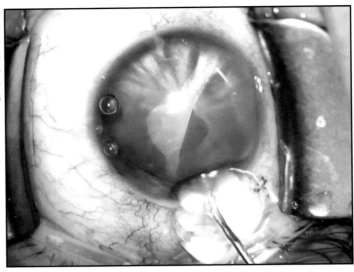

centesis, using a cystotome needle or small, 25-gauge microforceps, so that the chamber is closed and the anterior chamber pressure is maintained.

After the capsulorrhexis has started, gently rock the nucleus to release any intumescent fluid that may have been trapped between the posterior capsule and lens nucleus. If liquefied lens fluid is left between the posterior capsule and the lens nucleus, it can push the cataract anterior and exert force, which could radialize the capsulorrhexis. With this technique of decompressing the intracapsular pressure while maintaining an elevated anterior chamber pressure, we can complete a round capsulorrhexis in the majority of these white intumescent cataracts.

ANOTHER OPTION

Another option is to make a round opening, as it has no corners or weak spots that could radialize in the anterior lens capsule at once. This can be accomplished by using the phaco probe to punch out a disc from the anterior lens capsule, followed by decompression of the capsular bag, reinflation of the anterior chamber with viscoelastic, and then capsulorrhexis creation; alternatively, a femtosecond laser can be used to make the capsulorrhexis, as it would cut the entire capsule opening at once, with the anterior chamber pressurized with the suction ring.

NUCLEAR DENSITY

The nuclear density can vary greatly, with some white cataracts being soft, milky, and intumescent in nature (Figure 39-2), whereas others can be hard and rock-like, with a high degree of nuclear sclerosis (Figure 39-3). The differentiation between a dense white cataract and a soft white cataract is important in devising a surgical plan for phacoemulsification.

Dense white cataracts tend to be in patients age 65 and older. On slit-lamp examination, there is a yellow to brown hue to the central portion of the crystalline lens. The anterior capsule tends to look relatively flat, with no evidence of fluid within the capsular bag. After the capsule is stained with trypan blue dye, the capsulorrhexis should be fairly routine, with little risk of radialization. However, due to the density of the nucleus, a larger degree of ultrasonic phaco energy likely will be required, and the risk of corneal endothelial trauma or even phaco wound burn is higher. For these eyes, re-coating the endothelium with a dispersive viscoelastic during phaco and utilizing ultrasonic power modulations can help to lessen the risks.[2]

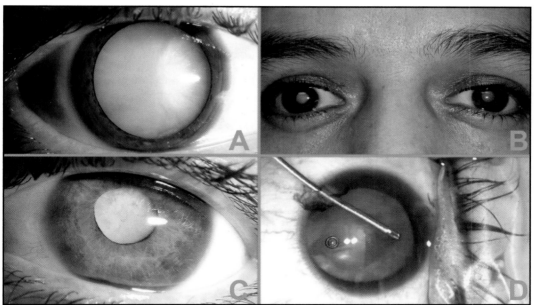

Figure 39-2. Soft, milky-white cataracts. These cataracts are liquid filled and pose additional challenges during surgery. (A) A homogenous, milky appearance of the entire lens (B) is more common in younger patients, who often present with bilateral cataracts. (C) The lack of any yellow or brown tones in the lens is indicative of less nuclear sclerosis. (D) Keeping the anterior chamber pressurized and using microforceps help to minimize complications during capsulorrhexis creation.

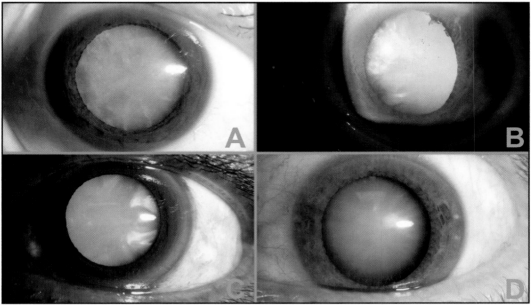

Figure 39-3. Dense white cataracts. These cataracts exhibit a significant degree of central nuclear opalescence and density, with very little of the milky, liquid appearance. (A) Note the yellow and brown tones in the lens centrally and (B, C) with cortical changes. (D) Sometimes the central nucleus is far more opaque than the peripheral area of the lens.

Conclusion

Most of the time, careful preoperative examination can identify challenges that can be addressed successfully during cataract surgery. Such patients tend to be among our very happiest, as they literally can go from blind to clear vision with our surgical techniques.

References

1. Chakrabarti A, Singh S. Phacoemulsification in eyes with white cataract. *J Cataract Refract Surg.* 2000;26(7):1041-1047.
2. Vajpayee RB, Bansal A, Sharma N, Dada T, Dada VK. Phacoemulsification of white hypermature cataract. *J Cataract Refract Surg.* 1999;25(8):1157-1160.

SECTION III

POSTOPERATIVE QUESTIONS

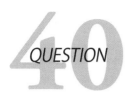

How Long Should Topical Antibiotics and Nonsteroidal Anti-Inflammatory Drugs Be Used Before and After Cataract Surgery?

Francis S. Mah, MD

First and foremost in the discussion of antibiotic prophylaxis for cataract surgery, it must be stressed that the use of the antiseptic povidone-iodine 5% solution in the conjunctival cul-de-sac prior to surgery is the cornerstone of endophthalmitis prophylaxis.

There is no consensus on which antibiotic to use or the method of application surrounding cataract surgery; however, there is general agreement that perioperative antibiotics are standard of care.[1]

Rationale for Using Preoperative and Postoperative Antibiotics

Because there are no prospective, randomized clinical trials regarding when to start antibiotic prophylaxis, we will defer to the plethora of studies performed by our general-surgery colleagues. The studies in general surgery have shown that the most efficacious time to use antibiotics are starting no more than 1 hour prior to surgery, with 30 minutes prior to incision being the optimal time to begin intravenous antibiotic prophylaxis.[2] Many ophthalmic surgeons point to studies done by Bucci[3] and Ta et al[4] showing a decrease in periocular bacterial flora as the rationale for using preoperative topical antibiotics for 1 to 7 days prior to cataract surgery.

Although this is surrogate evidence that there may be prophylactic efficacy to this strategy, other reasons may make this strategy useful; for example, teaching patients to use medications from a reusable dropperette. Because there is no extra cost to the health care system, one bottle typically lasts more than enough time for effective cataract surgery prophylaxis. As most likely there is no harm being done, as long as the patient is using the medication in the manner accepted by the US Food and Drug Administration (FDA); the strategy of using preoperative antibiotics 1 day or more prior to cataract surgery can be an acceptable means for prophylaxis, if not yet proven.

The reason I do not prescribe antibiotics for 1 or more days prior to surgery stems from my fear that the patient may not follow instructions, as they could typically be given weeks before surgery. If patients were to use the antibiotic for weeks prior to surgery, or use varying doses, resistant bacteria may be selected prior to surgery. Another issue may be that, if the patient did not use the antibiotics prior to surgery, does one cancel the surgery because the medication was not used? If not, the patient may question why it was recommended to be used in the first place. Furthermore, a patient may lose the bottle or use the entire bottle prior to surgery, adding to the cost of surgery.

Again, because the ophthalmic peer-reviewed literature is of no help in terms of the optimal time to end postoperative use of antibiotics for the purpose of prophylaxis, we will turn to the general-surgery literature, which shows that the benefits of postoperative intravenous antibiotics last for the first 12 hours and for a maximum of 24 hours.[5] The general feeling for ophthalmic surgery is to use topical antibiotics until the epithelium is healed, roughly 3 to 10 days.[1] Due to the use of topical steroids following cataract surgery, which are not typically used following general-surgery procedures, I think it is prudent to use topical antibiotics until the epithelium is intact following cataract surgery. Although it is typical to taper steroids and other anti-inflammatory medications, it is important not to taper antibiotics due to the real risk of selecting for resistent bacteria, thus developing new and more dangerous strains.[6]

Therefore, the recommendation is to use topical antibiotics starting at least 30 minutes to 1 hour prior to surgery and to continue the medication at full FDA dosages until the epithelium is healed, roughly 3 to 10 days, without tapering the antibiotic.

CHOOSING WHICH ANTIBIOTIC TO USE

Which antibiotic to use is even less clearly elucidated. Several caveats to keep in mind while deciding which antibiotic to use include peak concentrations (Cmax) in the ocular tissues and the minimum inhibitory concentration (MIC) of the key bacteria that cause endophthalmitis. Other characteristics may be considered, such as spectrum of coverage, cidal versus static mechanism of action, biocompatibility, and cost, but the main characteristics that define antibiotic efficacy are Cmax and MIC.

Today in ophthalmic surgery, fluoroquinolones have the combination of generally the lowest MICs and the highest concentrations in ocular tissues when used topically. Currently, among the fluoroquinolone class, besifloxacin, gatifloxacin, and moxifloxacin are the most potent (lowest MICs) and have the highest concentrations in the cornea and the anterior chamber (highest Cmax).[7] It is my opinion that cataract surgeons should be utilizing one of these 3 agents for perioperative cataract surgery prophylaxis. The choice also may vary depending on the resistance patterns in the area and the medical history of the patient, such as a history of methicillin-resistant *Staphylococcus aureus* colonization. The surgeon may wish to consult with the local infectious disease specialist to aid in choosing the best prophylactic antibiotic.

Should Antibiotic Use Become a Standard of Care?

Recently, many retrospective and prospective studies evaluating intracameral antibiotics injected at the conclusion of surgery have created earnest discussion among cataract surgeons regarding the future of prophylaxis. The published study findings report significant reduction in the rates of endophthalmitis when using intracameral antibiotics at the conclusion of surgery.[1] Intracameral antibiotics may be the future of cataract surgery endophthalmitis prophylaxis, but questions must be addressed before it should become the standard of care, including optimal drug, optimal dose, and potential short-term and long-term adverse effects of injecting such medications intracamerally.

Using Nonsteroidal Anti-Inflammatory Drugs

Unlike the use of topical antibiotics, the perioperative use of topical nonsteroidal anti-inflammatory drugs (NSAIDs) surrounding cataract surgery has been studied in prospective trials. Regarding miosis prevention, management of postoperative pain, and control of postoperative inflammation, the peer-reviewed literature is unanimous in reporting that topical NSAID use 3 days prior to surgery is superior to 1 day, which is superior to day of surgery.[8,9]

Postoperative length of therapy for an NSAID is less elucidated in the literature. The general opinion is that topical NSAID use should be for 3 or 4 weeks following cataract surgery, but this not based on efficacy studies.[8,9] If we look at the fact that cystoid macular edema (CME) has a peak incidence of 4 to 6 weeks following routine uncomplicated cataract surgery, then it makes sense that the NSAID should be used for at least 6 to 8 weeks after surgery to cover the high-risk period, with the understanding that no commercially available topical NSAID is approved for the prevention of CME. In those patients at high risk for CME, such as diabetics, uveitics, history of vasculopathy, and complicated surgery patients, to name a few, the use of prophylactic NSAIDs should be continued for at least 8 to 12 weeks after surgery. The dosing should never exceed the FDA-recommended frequency, and the NSAID should be monitored carefully in all patients with extended use beyond 2 weeks, due to the risk of corneal and scleral melts. The risk of these postoperative melts are highest in neurotrophic keratopathy patients, severe dry eye patients, and other patients with moderate to severe ocular surface disease, such as blepharitis and meibomitis.[8,9]

Regarding the NSAID of choice, the peer-reviewed literature shows the efficacy of diclofenac, ketorolac 0.5%, bromfenac 0.09%, nepafenac 0.1%, and nepafenac 0.3% in the management of postcataract surgery inflammation and pain.[10] Diclofenac, ketorolac, bromfenac, and nepafenac have been shown to be efficacious in the management of CME in the literature. In addition, nepafenac 0.1% has been shown to be effective in preventing diabetic macular edema postcataract surgery.[9] Newer NSAIDs, such as bromfenac and nepafenac, are reportedly more potent and more bioavailable after topical dosing than prior generations of NSAIDs. Nepafenac is the only pro-drug.[10]

Until there is prospective data showing differences between the available NSAIDs, it makes sense that the pain management, CME prevention, and anti-inflammatory efficacy are class effects. Several key differences are the dosing, once daily to 4 times daily; the formulations; solution versus suspension; and the rate of burning and stinging in the FDA trials of 0% to 40%.[11]

Conclusion

The recommendation for topical NSAID use for all patients undergoing cataract surgery, except for those mentioned at high risk for sclero-corneal melts, is 3 days optimally, day of surgery minimally, prior to cataract surgery at the FDA-approved dose and extended for 6 to 8 weeks following surgery. For those patients at high risk for CME following cataract surgery, the use of NSAIDs should begin at least 3 days prior to surgery and should continue for at least 8 to 12 weeks after surgery (Table 40-1).

Table 40-1
Topical Nonsteroidal Anti-Inflammatory Drugs and Dosing Regimen

Drug	Routine Patients	High Risk Patients
Diclofenac	QID for 4 to 6 weeks	QID for 6 to 12 weeks
Ketorolac 0.45%; 0.5%	QID for 4 to 6 weeks	QID for 6 to 12 weeks
Ketorolac 0.4%	BID for 4 to 6 weeks	BID for 6 to 12 weeks
Bromfenac 0.09%	BID for 4 to 6 weeks	BID for 6 to 12 weeks
Bromfenac 0.09%	QD for 4 to 6 weeks	QD for 6 to 12 weeks
Bromfenac 0.07%	QD for 4 to 6 weeks	QD for 6 to 12 weeks
Nepafenac 0.1%	TID for 4 to 6 weeks	TID for 6 to 12 weeks
Nepafenac 0.3%	QD for 4 to 6 weeks	QD for 6 to 12 weeks

References

1. Barry P, Seal DV, Gettinby G; ESCRS Endophthalmitis Study Group. ESCRS study of prophylaxis of postoperative endophthalmitis after cataract surgery: preliminary report of principal results from a European multicenter study [published correction appears in *J Cataract Surg.* 2006;32(5):709]. *J Cataract Refract Surg.* 2006;32(3):407-410.
2. Mangram AJ, Horan TC, Pearson ML, Silver LC, Jarvis WR. Guideline for prevention of surgical site infection, 1999. Hospital Infection Control Practices Advisory Committee. *Infect Control Hosp Epidemiol.* 1999;20(4):250-278.
3. Bucci FA Jr. An in vivo study comparing the ocular absorption of levofloxacin and ciprofloxacin prior to phaco-emulsification. *Am J Ophthalmol.* 2004;137(2):308-312.
4. Ta CN, He L, Nguyen E, De Kasper HM. Prospective randomized study determining whether a 3-day application of ofloxacin results in the selection of fluoroquinolone-resistant coagulase-negative *Staphylococcus. Eur J Ophthalmol.* 2006;16(3):359-364.
5. Bratzler DW, Houck PM. Antimicrobial prophylaxis for surgery: an advisory statement from the National Surgical Infection Prevention Project. *Clin Infect Dis* 2004;38(12):1706-1715.
6. Mah FS. Fourth-generation fluoroquinolones: new topical agents in the war on ocular bacterial infections. *Curr Opin Ophthalmol.* 2004;15(4):316-320.
7. Mah FS. The benefits of fourth generation fluoroquinolones in the prevention of ocular infections. *Clinical and Surgical Ophthalmology.* 2004;22(8):228-231.
8. O'Brien TP. Emerging guidelines for use of NSAID therapy to optimize cataract surgery patient care. *Current Medical Research and Opinion.* 2005;21(7):1131-1137.
9. Lindstrom R, Kim T. Ocular permeation and inhibition of retinal inflammation: an examination of data and expert opinion on the clinical utility of nepafenac. *Current Medical Research and Opinion.* 2006;22(2):397-404.
10. McColgin AZ, Heier JS. Control of intraocular inflammation associated with cataract surgery. *Curr Opin Ophthalmol.* 2000;11(1):3-6.
11. Silverstein SM, Cable MG, Sadri E. Once daily dosing of bromfenac ophthalmic solution 0.09% for postoperative ocular inflammation and pain. *Curr Med Res Opin.* 2011;27(9):1693-1703.

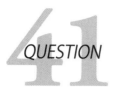

WHAT IS CAUSING LOW OR HIGH INTRAOCULAR PRESSURE IN MY POSTOPERATIVE PATIENT?

Richard A. Lewis, MD

The control of intraocular pressure (IOP) following cataract surgery is essential for an uncomplicated postoperative recovery. Intraocular pressure that is too low or too high may compromise the visual outcome. Avoiding this problem requires fastidious surgical technique. Who is at risk, how do we determine etiology, and what are the options for treating it is the focus of this chapter.

Elevated Intraocular Pressure Following Cataract Surgery

Postoperative fluctuation in IOP is a common problem following cataract surgery. This is a very transient problem in some patients, whereas in others it can be vision threatening. Although it is not always predictable who will have high IOP, some patients are at higher risk. In those patients, preventive measures instituted during surgery or immediately after the procedure are essential. Many patients can tolerate transient elevated IOP after cataract surgery; however, those with a history of glaucomatous cupping, compromised retinal vasculature, or corneal endothelial disease are vulnerable to complications, especially when the IOP is over 30 mm Hg.

The most common reason for elevated IOP after uncomplicated cataract surgery is retained viscoelastic that blocks the egress of aqueous through the trabecular meshwork.[1] This is a transient phenomenon that typically lasts for 24 to 36 hours. However, the extent of the IOP elevation can be dramatic and concerning. This problem is best avoided by careful irrigation and aspiration of the viscoelastic material at the conclusion of surgery. Intracameral cholinergic agents appear to be of limited use in blunting the pressure rise caused by retained viscoelastic.

Postoperatively, there are various options to normalize the IOP in this setting (Table 41-1). The most direct approach involves releasing viscoelastic and aqueous from the eye through

---

Table 41-1
Treatment for Elevated Pressure After Cataract Surgery

- Prophylaxis: remove viscoelastic at conclusion of surgery
- Burping of paracentesis incision
- Medications
  - Topical (alpha agonist [eg, apraclonidine] or beta blocker [eg, timolol]) or carbonic anyhydrase [eg, dorzolamide or brinzolamide])
  - Systemic (carbonic anhydrase inhibitor [eg, acetazolamide])

---

the paracentesis site, often referred to as burping the wound. This is performed in the examination room with the patient seated at the slit lamp. After checking the IOP, and with the eye topically anesthetized, I use a 30-gauge needle to carefully penetrate the paracentesis site to allow a few drops of aqueous and viscoelastic to escape the wound. Gentle pressure with the needle on the posterior lip of the entry site facilitates release. It should be noted that this technique must be avoided in any patient who suffered a complicated surgery to avoid vitreous prolapse into the anterior chamber with rapid pressure gradient changes.

A speculum is usually unnecessary. Burping the wound can be repeated as needed to achieve an IOP at the desired level. I apply a topical antibiotic immediately afterward. It is important to remember that releasing aqueous through the paracentesis site may reduce pressure only for a brief time. Applying topical hypotensive drops helps to maintain pressure reduction until the viscoelastic is completely gone.

Normalization of IOP after cataract surgery demands a fully functional outflow system. Patients with preexisting ocular hypertension, glaucoma, or compromised outflow are at risk for a postoperative pressure rise.[2] This may occur even following uncomplicated procedures because of surgical trauma and anterior segment inflammation. In these patients, it is useful to pretreat with aqueous suppressants at the conclusion of surgery to prevent the pressure rise. I recommend using aqueous suppressants, such as the alpha agonists (apraclonidine or brimonidine), beta-blockers (timolol), or carbonic anhydrase inhibitors (dorzolamide, brinzolamide, or oral acetazolamide). Sometimes, a combination of these hypotensive agents may be necessary. Outflow drugs, such as the prostaglandin analogues in particular, are less effective in the immediate postoperative setting because they require a more prolonged onset of action and may induce anterior segment inflammation. In those patients with glaucomatous cupping and visual field loss, or any patient who can ill-afford a marked postoperative pressure rise, combining cataract and glaucoma surgery may be recommended.

When considering the various causes of pressure elevation after cataract surgery, topical steroids are often suspected. However, steroids in the immediate postoperative period are rarely a cause of the pressure rise. Typically, a steroid-induced glaucoma requires 3 to 6 weeks of continuous dosing to elicit an IOP response. You should not see this in the immediate postoperative period.

Pressure problems should be anticipated in cataract patients following surgical complications, such as posterior capsular tears and vitreous loss with or without dropped lens fragments. The combination of prolonged surgery, inflammation, retained lens fragments, and modified intraocular-lens placement should be a red flag for potential IOP problems. Careful clean up of the anterior segment, with removal of the residual lens material and prolapsing vitreous, is important to avoid this problem as well as other complications.

Hypotensive medications following complicated cataract surgery are often ineffective at controlling IOP. Pars plana vitrectomy and lensectomy for a dropped nucleus and vitreous debris should be undertaken early in the postoperative period to control a persistently elevated IOP and to prevent other complications. However, do not assume that vitreous surgery alone will control the IOP for all such patients. Complicated cataract surgery impairs outflow facility, and these patients can develop prolonged pressure elevation. Filtering surgery may be necessary for definitive pressure control.

Low Intraocular Pressure Following Cataract Surgery

Low IOP after cataract surgery usually implies a wound leak from the paracentesis site or cataract wound. Findings might include a shallow anterior chamber and corneal folds. Seidel testing with a fluorescein strip will help to localize the site. A wound leak carries the risk of serious complications, including hypotony, inflammation, iris–corneal touch, and endophthalmitis. Reformation of the anterior chamber is important. This requires injecting balanced salt solution or viscoelastic into the anterior chamber, as well as proper closure of the cataract incision sites, using 10-0 nylon sutures to ensure it remains watertight.

Less common causes of hypotony following cataract surgery include an inadvertent formation of a cyclodialysis cleft during surgery, retinal pathology (ie, hole or tear), and uveitis with ciliary body shutdown. A detailed clinical examination, including gonioscopy and dilated retinal examination, should determine the cause and appropriate management.

Conclusion

High and low IOP after cataract surgery is not uncommon. Simple measures, including meticulous surgery, fluorescein staining of the corneal wounds, prophylactic medications in high-risk patients, and postoperative burping of a paracentesis incision, are useful to avoid pressure-related complications.

References

1. O'Brien PD, Ho SL, Fitzpatrick P, Power W. Risk factors for a postoperative intraocular pressure spike after phacoemulsification. *Can J Ophthalmol.* 2007;42(1):51-55.
2. Barak A, Desatnik H, Ma-Naim T, et al. Early postoperative intraocular pressure pattern in glaucomatous and nonglaucomatous patients. *J Cataract Refract Surg.* 1996;22(5):607-611.

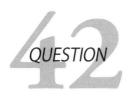
FOLLOWING UNEVENTFUL SURGERY, THREE OF MY EIGHT PATIENTS HAVE 4+ CELL AND FIBRIN ON POSTOPERATIVE DAY 1. WHAT SHOULD I DO?

Nick Mamalis, MD

Toxic Anterior Segment Syndrome

Toxic anterior segment syndrome (TASS) is an acute, sterile, postoperative anterior segment inflammation that can occur following cataract surgery.[1,2] It is not uncommon for TASS to occur in clusters, with several patients being affected on the same surgical day.

One of the hallmarks of TASS is that patients present with symptoms within 12 to 48 hours after surgery.

SYMPTOMS

It is very important to distinguish TASS from possible infectious endophthalmitis. The early onset is a helpful finding because symptoms in infectious endophthalmitis usually develop, on average, between 4 and 7 days postoperatively. In addition, although some patients may report pain, TASS patients are usually pain free, which is in contrast to infectious endophthalmitis in which up to 75% patients complain of pain. The most common clinical findings noted with TASS are marked anterior segment reaction, with increased cell and flare; hypopyon formation; and the possibility of fibrin on the surface of the intraocular lens within the pupillary space (Figure 42-1). In addition, widespread limbus-to-limbus corneal edema may be seen (Figure 42-2). Other findings may include damage to the iris, which may result in a dilated or irregular pupil, and damage to the trabecular meshwork, which can cause a delayed-onset glaucoma that is oftentimes difficult to treat (Figure 42-3).

CAUSES

The potential etiologic factors involved in TASS are extremely broad.[3] Problems with any of the solutions or medications that enter the eye during surgery can cause TASS. This includes balanced

Figure 42-1. Anterior segment inflammation with hypopyon formation.[3] (Reprinted from the *Journal of Cataract and Refractive Surgery,* 32/2, Mamalis N, Edelhauser HF, Dawson DG, Chew J, LeBoyer RM, Werner L, Toxic anterior segment syndrome, 324-333, 2006, with permission from Elsevier.)

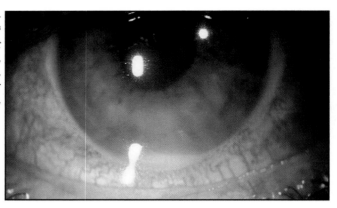

Figure 42-2. Diffuse limbus-to-limbus corneal edema.[3] (Reprinted from the *Journal of Cataract and Refractive Surgery,* 32/2, Mamalis N, Edelhauser HF, Dawson DG, Chew J, LeBoyer RM, Werner L, Toxic anterior segment syndrome, 324-333, 2006, with permission from Elsevier.)

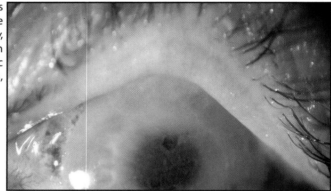

salt solution (BSS) or any additives placed in the BSS. One of the most common medications added to BSS is epinephrine. It is critical that the epinephrine be free of preservatives, including bisulfites. It is important that intracameral anesthetics, such as lidocaine, be preservative-free and injected in the proper dose. Intracameral antibiotics used any time during the surgery need to be prepared in the proper doses to ensure there is no chance of causing toxicity. Last, there have been cases of TASS secondary to ophthalmic ointment in the anterior segment of the eye following a clear corneal incision with tight patching, which may cause the wound to gape, allowing access of ointment into the eye.

Another important etiologic factor is the sterilization and preparation of instruments and tubing. Enzyme and detergent residues left on the instruments, especially inside of cannulas or handpieces, can cause toxicity. In addition, endotoxin residues may build up in ultrasound baths or water baths. Because they are heat-stable and survive autoclave sterilization, endotoxins remain on instruments and can cause intraocular inflammation if they are injected into the anterior segment of the eye.

It is critically important to ensure that all phacoemulsification and irrigation and aspiration handpieces, tips, and cannulas are thoroughly flushed at the conclusion of each surgery to make sure there is no residual ophthalmic viscosurgical device or cortex left within the lumens.

Careful evaluation of data provided from surveys and on-site visits of centers reporting cases of TASS to the American Society of Cataract and Refractive Surgery TASS Task Force showed that problems with instrument cleaning, especially inadequate flushing of ophthalmic instruments and handpieces, enzyme detergents, and ultrasound baths remain the most common factors. Data from the most recent 3-year period of analysis were compared with the previous 3-year data and found

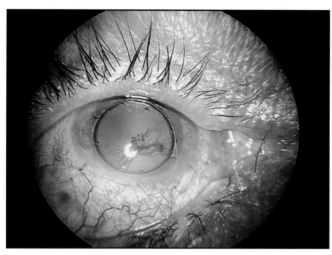

Figure 42-3. Dilated, atrophic iris with irregular pupil.[3] (Reprinted from the *Journal of Cataract and Refractive Surgery*, 32/2, Mamalis N, Edelhauser HF, Dawson DG, Chew J, LeBoyer RM, Werner L, Toxic anterior segment syndrome, 324-333, 2006, with permission from Elsevier.)

significant improvements in the percentage of sites using inadequate handpiece flushing volume, as well as the frequency of sites using an appropriate final rinse solution.[4] In addition, over this period of time, the frequency of TASS outbreaks declined and encouraging trends were seen in the use of reusable cannulas, as well as a decrease in the addition of antibiotics to BSS and use the of preserved intraocular medications. Overall, education may have helped to improve some instrument cleaning and perioperative practices that previously increased the risk of TASS; however, other practices were found to be headed in an unfavorable direction in this analysis.[4,5]

If a patient is suspected of having TASS, it is important to rule out an infectious etiology. The patient must undergo careful anterior segment evaluation, including slit lamp and gonioscopy. It is essential to assess the severity of the insult to the patient's anterior segment early in the course of his or her condition. The intraocular pressure should be monitored carefully because patients may initially have a low pressure that rapidly climbs secondary to damage to the trabecular meshwork.

TREATMENT

The mainstay of treatment for TASS is intense topical corticosteroids. These can include drops of prednisolone acetate 1% on an hourly basis initially. The patient should be followed very carefully during the first several days to ensure that the inflammation is improving during this period of time.

The clinical outcome is often dependent on the severity of the initial insult. Patients with a mild toxin exposure often will show rapid clearing of the inflammation in the anterior segment with little or no residual corneal or iris damage. However, patients with a more severe insult may have persistent corneal edema that may require a cornea transplant. Significant, persistent anterior segment inflammation may lead to problems with secondary glaucoma, pupillary and iris abnormalities, and cystoid macular edema.

Conclusion

As soon as an outbreak of TASS has been identified, it is critically important for the surgeon and all surgical center or hospital staff members to carefully review all protocols used in the cleaning and sterilization of instruments. It is important that the surgical staff is aware of the potential etiological factors involved with TASS and that all steps are taken to ensure that cannulas, handpieces, and other instruments are rinsed thoroughly with sterile, deionized water at the conclusion of each case. The use of detergents and enzymes within ultrasound baths should be evaluated carefully to ensure that residue is rinsed from all the instruments and that the water baths are being cleaned regularly and sterilized to ensure that there is no possibility for endotoxin contamination. Finally, a complete analysis of all medicines and fluids used during the surgery should be undertaken.

It is imperative for surgeons to be aware of the existence of TASS and the steps necessary to treat it to prevent future occurrences.

References

1. Monson MC, Mamalis N, Olson RJ. Toxic anterior segment inflammation following cataract surgery. *J Cataract Refract Surg.* 1992;18(2):184-189.
2. Mamalis N. Toxic anterior segment syndrome (Editorial). *J Cataract Refract Surg.* 2006;32(2):181-182.
3. Mamalis N, Edelhauser HF, Dawson DG, Chew J, LeBoyer RM, Werner L. Toxic anterior segment syndrome. *J Cataract Refract Surg.* 2006;32(2):324-333.
4. Bodnar Z, Clouser S, Mamalis N. Toxic anterior segment syndrome: update on the most common causes. *J Cataract Refract Surg.* 2012;38(11):1902-1910.
5. Cutler-Peck CM, Brubaker J, Clouser S, et al. Toxic anterior segment syndrome: common causes. *J Cataract Refract Surg* 2010;36(7):1073-1080.

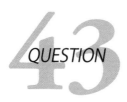

HOW DO I MANAGE HIGH-RISK UVEITIS PATIENTS PREOPERATIVELY AND POSTOPERATIVELY?

Michael B. Raizman, MD

Cataract extraction and lens implantation can be performed successfully in the majority of patients with uveitis, although special precautions are required to ensure a successful outcome. Coexisting conditions must be assessed and managed before surgery. These patients commonly have glaucoma, macular edema, vitreous debris, and epiretinal membranes. Lens implants might be avoided in certain patients with uveitis, such as children, adults with chronic granulomatous uveitis and extensive synechiae, and those with poorly controlled uveitis of any type; however, the majority of patients will tolerate and benefit from a lens implant.[1]

Treatment

Elimination of inflammation for at least 3 months before surgery is desirable. Flare may not be treatable, but cells in the anterior chamber should be extinguished. Prednisolone acetate or difluprednate drops should be used as often as needed prior to surgery. I continue these drops even after the cells are gone, up until the time of surgery. A typical patient will be on drops 2 to 4 times per day in the months leading up to surgery. Nearly all of my patients with uveitis receive a prophylactic course of oral prednisone around the time of surgery. If there are no systemic complications, I prescribe 60 mg daily beginning 3 days before surgery and continuing for approximately 7 days after surgery. The medication may be stopped without a taper, or it may be continued if there is excessive inflammation after surgery. Subconjunctival dexamethasone may be given during surgery as an alternative to oral therapy.

Synechiae can be lysed and the pupil can be stretched if necessary (Figure 43-1). Iris retractors or pupil-expansion devices can be helpful. The general goal is to minimize iris trauma as much as possible while allowing an adequate view for lens removal. I find a capsulorrhexis of 4 to 5 mm is ideal. If the rhexis is too large, posterior synechiae to the capsule edge after surgery can pull the

Figure 43-1. Eye with opaque cataract, posterior synechiae, and keratic precipitates following chronic uveitis.

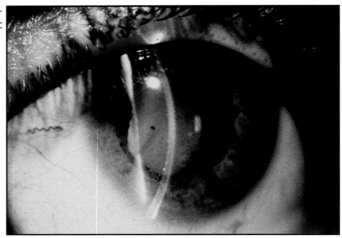

lens optic forward. Too small a rhexis can limit the view of the retina. Cataract removal may be combined with pars plana vitrectomy or trabeculectomy in selected cases.

More aggressive anti-inflammatory therapy than usual is required in many of these uveitic eyes. Applying drops every 1 to 2 hours in the first week is not usual, although difluprednate can be used less frequently than prednisolone acetate. Topical corticosteroid and nonsteroidal therapy may be continued for months, rather than weeks, and is titrated based on response to therapy. Intraorbital injection of steroids can be used for more severe inflammation. Cycloplegia need not be routine but should be considered in cases where fibrin is noted and the risk of pupillary block or synechiae formation appears likely. Systemic immunosuppression may be needed for those who required it before surgery and those who do not tolerate oral prednisone or have steroid-induced glaucoma.

What About Inflammation After Surgery in a Patient Who Did Not Have Uveitis Before Surgery?

Complicated surgery can lead to increased inflammation. Loss of vitreous, iris prolapse, intraoperative hemorrhage, iris stretching, iris damage, or corneal burns all can lead to unusual amounts of inflammation. Retention of lens fragments may be hard to diagnose. Gonioscopy, B-scan ultrasonography, and anterior segment ultrasound biomicroscopy or optical coherence tomography should be considered to look for retained material. Retained lens fragments in the anterior segment almost always should be removed surgically. These fragments may migrate and damage the corneal endothelium, leading to irreversible corneal edema. Uveitis and glaucoma from retained lens material are also concerns.

Intraocular lenses may stimulate uveitis if they are not ideally positioned. Mobile lenses are notorious for causing uveitis and cystoid macular edema. A haptic rubbing on the iris or ciliary body can cause inflammation. Anterior chamber lenses should be inspected for iris tuck or migration of a haptic through a peripheral iridectomy.

Excessive postoperative inflammation without prior iritis and without intraoperative complications can occur without warning. Treatment with topical corticosteroids should reduce or eliminate anterior chamber cells significantly.

Lack of response to topical therapy or the presence of significant vitreous inflammation should prompt the search for infection. Hypopyon, at any time after cataract surgery, should suggest infectious endophthalmitis. The capsular bag should be inspected closely for signs of abscess or plaques, but even a clear capsule may harbor bacteria. The presence of vitreal inflammation is always of concern. Any heightened suspicion should lead to a pars plana vitreous tap for culture and simultaneous injection of intravitreal antibiotics. This can be accomplished safely in the office. Broad-spectrum coverage can be achieved with intravitreal vancomycin and ceftazidime. In some cases, the posterior capsule must be opened to allow access of antibiotic to the capsular bag, where the organism is harbored. Yttrium aluminum garnet (YAG) capsulotomy or pars plana vitrectomy with capsulectomy may be of value prior to antibiotic treatment.

Inflammation may begin many months after cataract surgery in cases of low-grade endophthalmitis. Propionibacterium acnes is notorious for this, but it also may arise from staphylococcal, fungal, and other microbial infections.

Reference

1. Raizman MB. Cataract surgery in uveitis patients. In: Steinert RF, ed. *Cataract Surgery*. 3rd edition. Philadelphia, PA: Saunders Elsevier; 2010:305-309.

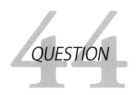

THE LENS HAS DROPPED. HOW SHOULD I MANAGE IT, AND WHEN SHOULD I REFER THE PATIENT TO A RETINA SPECIALIST?

Keith A. Warren, MD

Nothing is more anxiety provoking than when the expected rapidly turns to the unexpected. Perhaps nowhere else in ophthalmology do we generate more anxiety than when a supposed routine cataract procedure is complicated by capsular rupture and posterior dislocation of lens fragments. Although those fragments certainly may have been lost posteriorly, all is not lost. With proper management acutely and in the immediate postoperative period, patients can have excellent results, and the cataract surgeon has an important role perioperatively in helping the patient achieve a good final outcome.

Managing Complications

The key tenets for the successful management of surgical complications are the same across specialties. Be prepared, do not panic, perform a careful inspection, and stay within the comfort zone of your ability. Surgeons are experts at what they do most often. Trouble usually follows us when we move out of our comfort zones.

The first order of business in management of posterior lens dislocation is observation and inspection. While you are taking a minute to gather yourself, use that time to inspect the eye so you can make an accurate assessment of the situation and formulate a plan of action. Is there vitreous prolapse? Is there vitreous in the wound? How much of the lens is left anteriorly? What is the status of the capsule? How much of the lens fragment is lost posteriorly? Are the posterior fragments nuclear or cortical in nature? The answers to these questions are an integral part of an adequate assessment of the eye and should allow for the formulation of a clear plan of action.

TAGGING THE VITREOUS

The most reasonable first surgical maneuver is addressing the vitreous. Vitreous loss and lack of adequate cleanup usually is fraught with complications, including pupil irregularity, persistent inflammation, cystoid macular edema (CME), retinal tear, and retinal detachment. Clear identification of the location and extent of vitreous prolapse can be augmented by placement of triamcinolone acetonide (Kenalog) or Triesence (preservative-free triamcinolone acetonide) into the anterior chamber. The triamcinolone should be diluted prior to instillation. The surgeon can dilute the drug by adding 0.3 mL of triamcinolone to 0.7 mL of balanced salt solution. This 1-mL suspension then is added copiously into the anterior chamber, preferably through the paracentesis site, paying particular attention to the wound and angle. The triamcinolone then is irrigated from the anterior chamber with balanced salt solution. The particulate nature of the suspension does an excellent job of identifying and "labeling" the vitreous, and also may potentially provide some anti-inflammatory effect. After the vitreous has been "tagged" with triamcinolone, the anterior chamber should be, as described by Chang and others, "compartmentalized" with a dispersive viscoelastic such as Viscoat (sodium chondroitin sulfate; Alcon Laboratories) to segment the vitreous and remove it from the wound.[1-3] In addition, viscoelastic also can be used anteriorly to displace the lens fragments that remain in the capsule and iris plane for easier and safer removal. No attempt should be made to bring forward fragments that have dislocated posteriorly.

REMOVAL OF FRAGMENTS

After the vitreous has been identified and compartmentalized, removal may commence. The anterior vitrectomy should be performed bimanually, using a separate irrigation port and, preferably, a smaller-gauge cutter. These instruments should enter the anterior chamber through separate paracentesis sites as close to the 12-o'clock and 6-o'clock meridians as possible, to allow for full access to the temporal wound and chamber angle. The cutter speed preferably should be 800 cuts per minutes, or higher if possible, to allow for vitreous removal with minimal exertion of vitreous traction. The irrigation should be as low as possible to maintain the anterior chamber (bottle height, 20 to 25 cm; 1 to 2 mL/min), while minimizing anterior vitreous prolapse. Cutting should begin in the "tagged" vitreous, and policing of the wound and angle should be performed initially. Avoidance of the dispersive viscoelastic will assist in chamber maintenance and keep further vitreous prolapse to a minimum. Any vitreous around residual anterior lens fragments should be removed secondarily. After the vitreous has been removed from the anterior chamber and residual lens adequately, any residual lens fragments in the anterior chamber should be removed, either manually or by ultrasound, if the anterior chamber is free of vitreous. Extending the wound to accommodate a lens loop is an acceptable option that works well for larger fragments and may reduce the incidence of corneal decompensation.

MANAGING THE LENS

When the anterior chamber is cleared adequately of vitreous and lens fragments, attention should be directed to the status of the lens capsule. If the capsule can be salvaged, an attempt should be made to insert a lens into the posterior chamber, either sulcus or intracapsular. In the absence of adequate capsular support, an anterior chamber lens or iris-sutured lens should be placed. Several studies in the literature suggest that final visual outcomes are best in complicated cataract surgery when the intraocular lens is placed at the time of initial surgery.[4] It should be noted that because these patients are at moderate risk for additional retinal complications, silicone lens implants should be avoided if possible in this setting.

ANTI-INFLAMMATORY TREATMENT

After the anterior segment has been policed and a lens implant has been placed, the anterior segment surgeon's job (the most important one) is nearly completed. Aggressive anti-inflammatory treatment for these patients to lower their risk of secondary complications, particularly CME, is recommended. A periocular injection of triamcinolone (20 mg per 0.5 mL of suspension) into the conjunctival cul-de-sac provides an excellent anti-inflammatory effect. In addition, a potent topical steroid and nonsteroidal anti-inflammatory should be administered at least 4 times per day in this patient population.

Conclusion

The indications for the removal of residual lens fragments in the posterior segment are as follows: media opacity obscuring the visual axis, intraocular inflammation, and glaucoma. It should be noted that, with adequate cleanup of the anterior segment and placement of a lens implant, the literature reports a lower incidence of secondary glaucoma and CME with improved final visual outcomes.[5] With regard to the timing of removal of the lens fragments by planned pars plana vitrectomy, no difference was noted between immediate removal or delayed removal regarding final visual outcomes when the removal occurred before 30 days.[6] The average time reported for planned removal was 15 days after initial surgery. Poor visual outcomes were more likely in eyes with poor presenting visual acuity, previtrectomy CME, retinal detachment, or delay in fragment removal beyond 30 days. The most common complication associated with vision loss was CME.[7] Despite this surgical complication, most patients have a favorable outcome, with the vast majority patients achieving 20/40 or better.

In summary, patients suffering from retained lens fragments following complicated surgery are best managed by cleanup of the anterior segment and placement of an intraocular lens at the initial surgery. Removal of the lens fragments before 1 month by planned vitrectomy usually results in excellent visual outcomes. Most complications are related to poor vitreous management and can be avoided with careful anterior segment cleanup and minimizing vitreous traction. Although this is a stressful event for all involved, most patients can have a favorable result.

Acknowledgements

I would like to acknowledge David F. Chang, MD (viscodispersive agents); David Boyer, MD (vitrectomy complications); and William Mieler, MD (timing of vitrectomy) for their contributions to this chapter.

References

1. Chang DF, Packard RB. Posterior assisted levitation for nucleus retrieval using Viscoat after posterior capsule rupture. *J Cataract Refract Surg.* 2003;29(10):1860–1865.
2. Chang DF. Managing Residual Lens Material after Posterior Capsule Rupture. *Techniques in Ophthalmology.* 2003;1(4):201–206.
3. Chang DF. Strategies for Managing Posterior Capsular Rupture. In: Chang DF, ed. *Phaco Chop: Mastering Techniques, Optimizing Technology, and Avoiding Complications.* Thorofare, NJ: Slack Incorporated; 2004:203-223.

4. Rofagha S, Bhisitkul RB. Management of retained lens fragments in complicated cataract surgery. *Curr Opin Ophthal.* 2011;22(2):137-140.
5. Scott IU, Flynn HW Jr, Smiddy WE, et al. Clinical features and outcomes of pars plana vitrectomy in patients with retained lens fragments. *Ophthalmology.* 2003;110(8):1567-1572.
6. Colyer MH, Berinstein DM, Khan NJ, et al. Same-day versus delayed vitrectomy with lensectomy for the management of retained lens fragments. *Retina.* 2011;31(8):1534-1540.
7. Cohen SM, Davis A, Cukrowski C. Cystoid macular edema after pars plana vitrectomy for retained lens fragments. *J Cataract Refract Surg.* 2006;32(9):1521-1526.

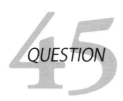

How Should I Manage a Postoperative Refractive Surprise?

Stephen S. Lane, MD

A postoperative refractive surprise is one of the most frustrating consequences of uncomplicated cataract surgery. When this occurs, the desired refractive result has not been achieved, leading most often to a patient who complains of poor uncorrected visual acuity. Prior to attempting to manage the problem, it is critical for the surgeon to determine the cause of the postoperative "surprise."[1] By determining causation, the best management can be planned.

Potential Etiologies

Potential etiologies for a postoperative refractive surprise would include measurement errors in either the axial length or keratometry readings; patients who have had previous refractive surgery, either known or unknown, prior to surgery; incorrect positioning of the intraocular lens (IOL); calculations errors; irregular astigmatism; and unidentified corneal ectasia due to keratoconus, form fruste keratoconus, pellucid marginal degeneration, or post laser in situ keratomileusis (LASIK) or photorefractive keratectomy (PRK) ectasia. Toric IOLs may have been placed off axis from lens rotation or an error may have been made in identification of the proper axis for the lens to be placed. Identification of the etiology for the refractive surprise will aid the surgeon in determining the best treatment.

Correcting Errors

Under most circumstances, if the etiology can be determined, the best treatment would be to remedy the error, if possible. For example, a misalignment of a toric IOL usually would be best served in rotating the lens to the proper position rather than performing a corneal refractive procedure.

It is important to understand that prevention certainly trumps any type of postoperative treatment. In this respect, accurate biometry and keratometry are necessary to avoid IOL power errors. It is also important to avoid the wrong IOL power, which can occur during a mixup in the operating room procedures. A "pause" before each procedure to reconfirm IOL power and the correct eye on which to operate is an important component of modern-day cataract surgery and can help to avoid the placement of an IOL that was not intended.

Minimization of surgically induced astigmatism by performing meticulous surgery is also a key factor. Compromise, such as in a corneal phaco wound burn, not only will disturb wound integrity greatly, but it also will induce signifcant astigmatism. Finally, when using IOLs, it is critical that the axis be identified correctly and the lens placed in the proper orientation.

MANAGEMENT STRATEGIES

Unfortunately, despite diligent adherence to the principles mentioned, refractive errors and IOL surprises still do occur. Management strategies include four alternatives:

1. Intraocular lens exchange
2. Incisional corneal refractive surgery, such as a peripheral corneal-relaxing incision for astigmatism
3. Laser corneal refractive surgery, including LASIK and PRK
4. The use of a piggyback IOLs

In addition to the potential etiologies discussed previously, a number of other factors are important to consider:

- The patient's age and general health are important. Can this patient tolerate another intraocular procedure, such as an IOL exchange or a piggyback IOL?

- What is the nature of the patient's complaint? Is the complaint consistent with the residual refractive error? If not, close observation, rather than performing a procedure, might be indicated.

- What is the length of time following surgery? Might the problem, such as a toric IOL off axis that needs to be rotated, "settle out" over time, or should it be handled more urgently?

- What is the nature of the residual refractive error? Is it spherical or cylindrical? Is there irregular astigmatism that may not be helped significantly by an intraocular procedure?

- What does the patient's topography look like, and does the macula appear normal with optical coherence tomography testing?

- What is the position and condition of the IOL in the capsule? Certainly, any compromise to the capsule or IOL would suggest that an extraocular procedure, such as corneal laser vision correction, be considered because of the potential complications associated with intraocular surgery in the presense of an open posterior capsule.[2]

- Most importantly, can the error be cured with spectacle correction? If it cannot, conditions such as cystoid macular edema, corneal irregularity, or optic nerve compromise must be considered. In most IOL surprise cases, given an uncomplicated surgical procedure, correction of the refractive error should allow the patient to attain excellent vision in an otherwise normal eye.

The following cases will demonstrate those instances where one alternative might be preferred over another.

CASE 1

Postoperatively, the patient is unhappy with uncorrected visual acuity of 20/40 that improves to better than 20/20, with a residual refraction of –0.75 +1.50 x 90, 2 months after surgery. The remainder of the examination is entirely normal, and the opposite eye is plano with 20/20 vision.

Solution: In my opinion, this patient would be best served with a peripheral corneal-relaxing incision at axis 90 degrees. Notice that the spherical equivalent in this patient is plano; therefore, as a result of coupling, a peripheral corneal-relaxing incision or a pair of peripheral corneal-relaxing incisions should relieve the astigmatism, as well as the residual myopia, leaving this patient essentially plano.

CASE 2

A 60-year-old patient, status post LASIK, underwent uncomplicated cataract surgery. Despite a target of plano, an IOL surprise occurred, leaving the patient with a –3.00-diopter (D) sphere correction noted 1 week after surgery. There was no change in the refractive error after 3 months, and vision continued to correct to 20/20 with a –3.00-D sphere correction.

Solution: This otherwise healthy patient can certainly tolerate an intraocular procedure and thus would be best served, in my opinion, with an IOL exchange. While performing LASIK (PRK would be another possible solution), the results could be compounded by the previous corneal refractive procedure that preceded cataract surgery. This problem, when recognized shortly (approximately 6 weeks) after surgery, allows for relatively easy surgical removal and exchange of the lens with one that can be predictably calculated.

CASE 3

An 80-year-old enthusiastic reader with long-standing emphysema and on oxygen is referred for difficulty in using both eyes together. Previous cataract surgery in the right eye left a residual refractive error of –1.50 D sphere with 20/20 acuity. Cataract surgery, performed 8 months prior in the left eye, has left the patient with a residual refractive error of +3.00 D sphere and 20/20 acuity. He is having difficulty using both eyes together and is bothered particularly when he attempts to read. The IOL in each eye is in perfect position within the capsular bag, and the posterior capsule is intact. The examination is normal otherwise.

Solution: The best solution for this patient, in my opinion, would be a piggyback IOL in the left eye. Although an IOL exchange is possible, after 3 months there may be significant adherence of the lens within the capsular bag, and the potential for compromise of the capsule in IOL removal is a distinct possibility. Given that the patient has significant emphysema, I would want to spend as little time as possible performing intraocular surgery. A piggyback IOL can be calculated easily, using a vergence formula, and placed in the ciliary sulcus for this gentleman. Although a corneal refractive procedure could be entertained, the possibility of a poor ocular surface in an 80-year-old patient should be considered, as it could lead to delayed wound healing and visual rehabilitation.

CASE 4

A patient who had uncomplicated surgery with multifocal IOL implantation presents to you with an uncorrected distance visual acuity at distance of 20/50 at 6 months after surgery. He is dissatisfied with this level of uncorrected visual acuity. The residual refractive error is –1.75 +0.75 x 90. The lens is in good position within the lens capsule. The examination is otherwise unremarkable, with normal pachymetry and regular topography.

Solution: This is an ideal patient for corneal laser refractive surgery, either LASIK or PRK, depending on the surgeon's preference. An IOL exchange alone would not resolve the residual cylinder without accompanying peripheral corneal-relaxing incisions. The predictability of such a combination of procedures, in my experience, is not as accurate as with a corneal refractive procedure.

Conclusion

The demands of today's cataract patients continue to increase. As a result, ophthalmic surgeons must be prepared to manage residual refractive errors and IOL surprises following uneventful cataract surgery. The identification of the etiology of the error and utilization of modalities discussed should be a part of the modern cataract surgeon's armamentarium.

References

1. Mamalis N. Complications of foldable intraocular lenses requiring explantation or secondary intervention—2007 survey update. *J Cataract Refract Surg.* 2008;34(9):1584-1591.
2. Hayashi K, Hirata A, Hayashi H. Possible predisposing factors for in-the-bag and out-of-the-bag intraocular lens dislocation and outcomes of intraocular lens exchange surgery. *Ophthalmology.* 2007;114(5):969-975.

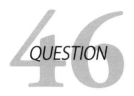

WHAT CAUSES MY PATIENTS TO COMPLAIN ABOUT TEMPORAL SHADOWS OR REFLECTIONS, AND HOW SHOULD I MANAGE PERSISTENT SYMPTOMS?

Samuel Masket, MD and
Nicole R. Fram, MD

Dysphotopsias, both negative and positive, although diverse in cause and cure, represent undesired optical phenomena following cataract surgery. They interfere significantly with quality of vision and the perceived success of surgery. In reality, dysphotopsia represents a failure of both the manufacturing sector and the clinician in recognizing and correcting the matter. Presently, dysphotopsia accounts for the greatest incidence of patient dissatisfaction after otherwise uncomplicated cataract surgery, and its importance has been overlooked greatly. Given that negative dysphotopsia (ND) and positive dysphotopsia (PD) differ in etiology and management, they will be considered separately. However, both conditions may exist simultaneously.

Negative Dysphotopsia

Negative dysphotopsia was originally described by Davison as complaints of a dark temporal crescent, similar to horse blinders.[1] Clinical experience dictates that there are no beneficial medical therapies for the patient with symptomatic ND. However, surgical methods have been devised that have proved to be useful in reducing ND visual symptoms. Although ND rarely induces visual disability sufficient to require an operative approach, some patients are very disturbed by it and can be very vocal in their complaints. This may be particularly true when premium intraocular lenses (IOLs) have been implanted.

Perhaps the most frustrating aspect of this problem for the surgeon and patient alike is that ND occurs only in cases of what we consider to be perfect surgery. That is, ND has been reported only in cases where the posterior chamber IOL (PC IOL) is well-centered within the confines of the capsular bag. To our understanding, ND has never been reported with sulcus-placed PC IOLs or anterior chamber IOLs. In our investigation, we found that ND occurs with any type

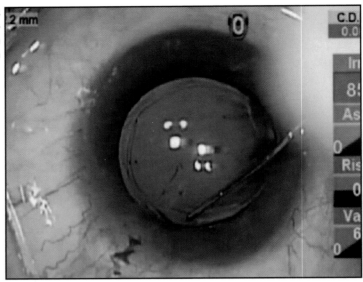

Figure 46-1. A Sinskey hook is fed underneath the anterior capsule following viscodissection in an attempt to free the optic from the capsule.

of in-the-bag PC IOLs, with overlap of the anterior capsulorrhexis onto the anterior surface of the PC IOL.[2] Fortunately, symptoms are transient in most cases.

REVERSE OPTIC CAPTURE

Given the above, and in keeping with our studies, 2 surgical strategies have emerged as beneficial for patients with chronic symptoms: reverse optic capture (ROC) and placement of a secondary piggyback IOL. Failed surgical strategies include within-the-bag IOL exchange, wherein the original implant is removed and another IOL of different material, shape, or edge design is replaced within the capsular bag. This is in keeping with the work of Vamosi et al.[3]

Reverse optic capture may be used in a secondary surgery for symptomatic patients or as a primary prophylactic strategy. In cases of the latter, the method has been applied to the second eye of patients who were significantly symptomatic following routine, uncomplicated surgery in their first eye. It should be noted, however, that ND symptoms are not necessarily bilateral.

Secondary ROC, performed for symptomatic patients, may be applied if the anterior capsulotomy is not too small, too thick, or rigid from postoperative fibrosis. At surgery, the anterior capsule is freed from the underlying optic by gentle, blunt dissection and viscodissection (Figure 46-1). Next, the nasal anterior capsular edge is retracted with one Sinskey hook (Bausch & Lomb Inc) or a similar device, while the optic edge is elevated and the capsular edge is allowed to slip under the optic (Figure 46-2). This maneuver is repeated 180 degrees away temporally, leaving the haptics undisturbed in the bag (Figures 46-3, 46-4, and 46-5).

Primary or prophylactic ROC is performed at the time of initial cataract surgery for the symptomatic patient's fellow eye. It should be recognized that surgical success in achieving primary or secondary ROC is highly dependent on a properly sized and centered anterior capsulorrhexis. There seems to be little optical consequence of ROC, as the haptics remain in the bag; theoretically, however, a modest myopic shift would be induced, varying directly with the power of the IOL.

PIGGYBACK INTRAOCULAR LENS

The other surgical method that has proved to be successful for patients with symptomatic ND is a piggyback IOL, as first reported by Ernest.[4] In this method, a second IOL is implanted in

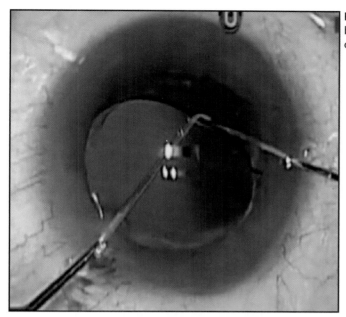

Figure 46-2. The Sinskey hook and blunt spatula are used to elevate the optic edge over the capsule.

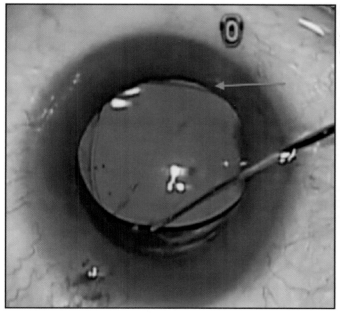

Figure 46-3. After the nasal edge has been captured (arrow), the opposite, temporal edge of the optic is elevated over the anterior capsular edge.

the ciliary sulcus atop the existing IOL and capsule bag complex. It appears that covering the primary optic and capsular junction reduces ND symptoms, although the original concept was that a piggyback lens was effective because it collapsed the posterior chamber by reducing the distance between the posterior iris and the anterior surface of the IOL. However, our studies have determined that the depth of the posterior chamber is unrelated to ND symptoms.[2] We prefer use of a 3-piece silicone IOL. Regarding ametropia, for hyperopic errors, multiply the spectacle error by 1.50 diopters (D) to determine IOL power, whereas for myopic errors multiply by 1.20 D. For example, in the case of a 2.00-D hyperopic patient, implant a +3.00-D IOL in the ciliary sulcus.

Figure 46-4. Optic capture has been completed. The nasal and temporal edges of the implant are anterior to the anterior capsule (arrows), whereas the haptics remain fully within the capsular bag.

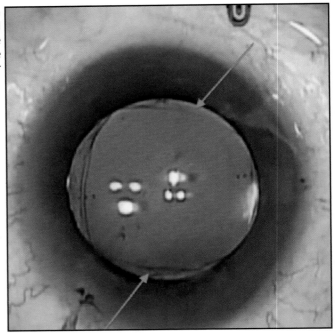

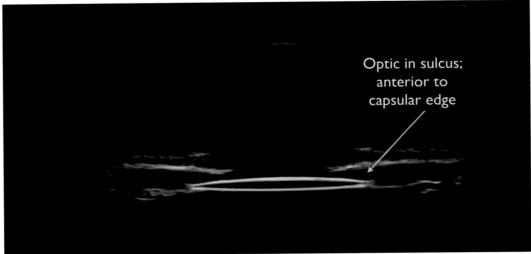

Optic in sulcus; anterior to capsular edge

Figure 46-5. Ultrasound biomicroscopy demonstrating reverse optic capture with the optic edge anterior to the capsular edge.

Positive Dysphotopsia

Positive dysphotopsia is reported by patients as light streaks, halos, starbursts, and so forth. It may be induced by internal reflections from either the optic edge or the optic surfaces.[5] Therefore, PD appears to be related directly to IOL material, optic size, index of refraction, radius of curvature, surface reflectivity, and edge design. Typically, PD is associated with a thick, square-edged design, high index of refraction, low radius of curvature, and high surface reflectivity.[6,7]

Unlike ND, patients may perceive benefit from use of miotic agents, particularly under dim light conditions. Medical management of PD includes brimonidine tartrate 0.15%, which can be tried initially. Also useful is a dilute solution of pilocarpine, typically 0.5%. Athough topical miotics may be helpful, they are associated with the potential for allergies and side effects.

Should miotic therapy prove unsuccessful and the symptoms mandate further treatment, IOL exchange may be highly successful. In this situation, opt for a lens with a low index of refraction, large optic diameter, and a thin, round-edged design.

Conclusion

Patients with either ND or PD require careful, concerned attention to their symptoms and a meaningful discussion of the suspected etiology, and they should be presented with a supportive plan for assistance.

References

1. Davison JA. Positive and negative dysphotopsia in patients with acrylic intraocular lenses. *J Cataract Refract Surg.* 2000;26(9):1346-1355.
2. Masket S, Fram NR. Pseudophakic negative dysphotopsia: surgical management and new theory of etiology. *J Cataract Refract Surg.* 2011;37(7):1199-1207.
3. Vamosi P, Csákány B, Németh K. Intraocular lens exchange in patients with negative dysphotopsia symptoms. *J Cataract Refract Surg.* 2010;36(3):418-424.
4. Ernest PH. Severe photic phenomenon. *J Cataract Refract Surg.* 2006;32(4):685-686.
5. Holladay JT, Lang A, Portney V. Analysis of edge glare phenomena in intraocular lens edge designs. *J Cataract Refract Surg.* 1999;25(6):748-752.
6. Masket S. Truncated edge design, dysphotopsia, and inhibition of posterior capsule opacification. *J Cataract Refract Surg.* 2000;26(1):145-147.
7. Masket S, Geraghty E, Crandall AS, et al. Undesired light images associated with ovoid intraocular lenses. *J Cataract Refract Surg.* 1993;19(6):690-694.

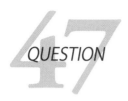

What Should I Do With the Unhappy Patient After Implantation of a Presbyopia-Correcting Intraocular Lens in One Eye? After Implantation in Two Eyes?

William Trattler, MD and
Gaston O. Lacayo III, MD

Presbyopic intraocular lenses (IOLs) have gained popularity among both patients and surgeons over the past few years. This can be attributed to improved technology, as well as improved pre-operative diagnostic testing, to help with appropriate lens selection for the patient.[1] However, even with careful preoperative screening, patients who undergo presbyopic IOL implantation can report dissatisfaction with their postoperative visual results, following surgery in both eyes or even after surgery in one eye. Being prepared to troubleshoot the causes that produce an unhappy presbyopic patient is critical to keeping an unhappy patient confident that their situation can be addressed and potentially solved.

Identifying Causes of Patient Dissatisfaction

Regardless of whether a patient reports dissatisfaction following surgery in 1 or both eyes, the initial steps to determine the underlying cause for the complaints are the same. A thorough history should be performed to determine if the complaint is due to inadequate distance, intermediate, or near vision, or whether the complaint is related to quality of vision issues such as glare or starbursts. Uncorrected vision should be checked at distance, intermediate, and near, along with refraction. The cornea, ocular surface, posterior capsule, optic nerve, and macula should be examined. Corneal topography, optical coherence tomography of the macula, and wavefront testing also should be performed to further help with the analysis of the source of the dissatisfaction.

The 2 most common reasons for an unhappy patient after presbyopic IOL implantation are ocular surface disease and residual refractive error, especially with patients who have 0.75 diopters or more of astigmatism.[1] If ocular surface disease is present, it should be addressed. Effective treatments include topical steroids, topical cyclosporine (Restasis; Allergen Inc), and insertion of punctual plugs if the ocular surface disease is due primarily to aqueous deficiency. For ocular surface disease related to meibomian gland dysfunction, use warm compresses, good eyelid hygiene, topical steroids, and topical azithromycin (Azasite; Merck). After the ocular surface disease is treated effectively, patients should return for repeat testing to determine whether their vision or visual complaints have improved or resolved.

For unhappy patients with a healthy ocular surface, it is important not to rely solely on the manifest refraction to determine whether the patient has residual astigmatism that has an impact on his or her vision. Topography may reveal more astigmatism than is present in the refraction, as well as mild-to-moderate residual astigmatism. Therefore, topography is a very important test to help to determine the underlying cause for a patient who is not satisfied with his or her vision.

Treatment Options

If residual refractive error is diagnosed and the ocular surface is healthy, the most effective way to improve the patient's situation is with some form of surgery to improve their uncorrected vision. For cases of myopia or hyperopia and low levels of astigmatism, surgeons can consider surface ablation, laser in situ keratomileusis (LASIK), or a piggyback IOL. If there is a combination of astigmatism and either myopia or hyperopia, surface ablation or LASIK can be performed. In some cases, implantation of a piggyback IOL with relaxing corneal incisions to address the astigmatism may be appropriate. Occasionally, patients have mixed astigmatism with a spherical equivalent close to plano, and relaxing corneal incisions with either a diamond blade or a femtosecond laser can be effective. By significantly reducing the residual refractive error and improving the uncorrected vision, patients often report a significant improvement in satisfaction.

An often-overlooked condition that leads to significant compromise of visual quality in presbyopic IOL patients is epithelial basement membrane dystrophy (map-dot-fingerprint dystrophy). The easiest way to identify this condition is to place fluorescein stain on the cornea, and, if present, areas of irregular epithelium will be revealed. This condition can be treated easily with epithelial debridement. Some surgeons prefer phototherapeutic keratectomy, whereas others prefer using a diamond burr to gently smooth the underlying stroma. After the condition has been treated, patients often experience significant improvement in visual quality.

Besides evaluating for residual refractive error, it is also critical to evaluate the corneal topography carefully to ensure there is no irregular astigmatism. This is especially important in patients with previous corneal refractive surgery because they can have a variety of abnormal corneal shapes, including a small optical zone, a decentered optical zone, or early ectasia, that will reduce the success of a presbyopic IOL. In these cases, laser vision correction or a piggyback IOL cannot solve their corneal condition, and an IOL exchange to monofocal vision may be the best option.

In patients where an IOL exchange to a monofocal implant is required, it obviously is easiest to perform the exchange in cases where the posterior capsule is intact. However, even if a yttrium aluminum garnet (YAG) capsulotomy has been performed, an IOL exchange is very straightforward. After the appropriate monofocal IOL power has been determined, the procedure is performed easily under topical anesthesia. A dispersive viscoelastic is placed into the capsular bag with the goal of freeing up the multifocal optic and haptics. The IOL usually can be rotated out of the bag without much difficulty. If the haptics cannot be liberated from the capsule, they can be amputated and left in place. The IOL can be removed through a small incision, either by folding it in the anterior chamber or by cutting it in half with IOL cutters, or it can removed through a larger incision. Some surgeons recommend placing the new IOL in the capsular bag prior to removing the original IOL. If the capsule is open, the main difference is that the new IOL should be 3-piece and placed in the sulcus and, if possible, the optic can be positioned through the rhexis (reverse optic capture).

Conclusion

It is important to carefully troubleshoot the reasons that a patient is dissatisfied with their presbyopic IOL implant. In the majority of cases, performing extensive testing, including topography, wavefront, optical coherence tomography of the macula, fluorescein staining of the cornea, and careful refraction, often can reveal the underlying reason for the complaints. Therapeutic options exist for virtually all conditions that lead to an unhappy presbyopic IOL patient, and, in most cases, definitive treatment can be performed for improvement.

Reference

1. Cillino S, Casuccio A, Di Pace F, et al. One-year outcomes with new-generation multifocal intraocular lenses. *Ophthalmology.* 2008;115(9):1508-1516.

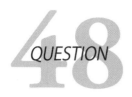

Following a Posterior Capsular Rent, the Sulcus-Fixated Intraocular Lens Has Become Decentered. How Should I Proceed?

Garry P. Condon, MD

Cause and Prevention

Intraocular lens (IOL) decentration is a common and often puzzling problem that occurs days to years after attempted IOL placement in the sulcus due to a posterior capsular tear. In the presence of an intact anterior capsulorrhexis, possible causes for decentration include inadequate IOL length for a large sulcus diameter, a localized zonular defect, haptic damage, or haptic memory loss. With a discontinuous capsulorrhexis, the subluxation of the IOL often may be caused by asymmetric bag or sulcus haptic positions aggravated by late contraction of the residual capsular complex. In either case, associated vitreous prolapse or incarceration can contribute to the IOL malposition and can cause a pupil deformity.

The intraoperative duress of dealing with a posterior capsular rent often clouds our thinking to the degree that we are happy simply to get the IOL in the sulcus. However, we usually can prevent subsequent IOL decentration by prolapsing the optic posteriorly through an intact anterior capsulorrhexis to capture it, while leaving the haptics in the sulcus. The importance of this simple maneuver cannot be overemphasized because it also prevents vitreous prolapse and pigment dispersion caused by the optic chafing the iris.

Treatment Options

I recommend intervention for a decentered IOL primarily for intolerable visual symptoms. Indications include reduced visual acuity, glare, edge-effect halos, and photophobia, as well as complications such as uveitis-glaucoma-hyphema syndrome and cystoid macular edema.[1] The intervention options include observation, miotics, or surgery with repositioning, exchange, or

Figure 48-1. A 23-gauge microforceps is used to grasp and manipulate a dislocated IOL.

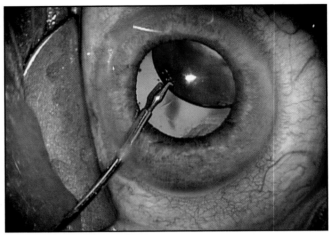

explantation of the IOL. Many of these IOLs remain in a mildly decentered but stable location, requiring only observation. I have found patient-directed miotic therapy with 1% pilocarpine to be useful for mild decentration that often is symptomatic only at night. In those patients needing surgical therapy for an out-of-the-bag decentered IOL, I prefer simple repositioning or peripheral iris suture fixation of the haptics. I reserve IOL exchange as a last option.

Preoperative Evaluation

The preoperative evaluation must include a detailed slit-lamp examination in an attempt to determine the position of the IOL in relation to any residual capsular layers. Preoperative gonioscopy may enhance visualization further. However, I often find it impossible to determine the amount of available capsular support and its degree of continuity until I am in the operating room, where I am able to retract the iris for an optimal view. Predilated and postdilated examinations best reveal iris anatomy and pupil function and whether there is the need to perform a pupilloplasty as part of the surgery.

Although sometimes difficult, it is important to determine the material and design of the decentered IOL. A large, single-piece poly (methyl methacrylate) (PMMA) IOL may be best suited to scleral fixation, as opposed to a 3-piece design with flexible haptics, which I prefer suturing to the iris. I attempt to obtain the original IOL power and routinely include biometry in evaluating all of these cases, as unanticipated IOL exchange is always a possibility.

Instrumentation

For simple repositioning or suture fixation, a small diamond knife enables me to make paracenteses without deforming the globe. Although a Sinskey hook (Bausch & Lomb Inc), a Kuglen hook (Katena Products Inc), and an iris spatula are all valuable, I find the recently available anterior segment microforceps from MicroSurgical Technologies Inc dramatically improves my ability to manipulate the IOL, iris, and capsule during surgery (Figure 48-1). Disposable nylon iris retractors are invaluable devices, not only to improve visualization while suturing but also to support the IOL haptic itself during fixation. I prefer viscoelastic agents, such as sodium hyaluronate (Healon; Abbott Medical Optics Inc or PROVISC; Alcon Laboratories), that are easy to remove completely through small incisions with simple irrigation. This reduces the risk of postoperative intraocular pressure elevation. The suture material I use for iris fixation is 10-0 polypropylene, threaded on a long, curved needle, such as the PC-7 (Alcon Laboratories), the CIF-4 (Ethicon), or the CTC-6 (Ethicon). I use 9-0 polypropylene for scleral fixation.

Surgical Techniques

The first question to consider before surgery is how widely the pupil should be dilated. Although mydriasis improves our view of the IOL position and available support, I often want to create temporary pupillary capture of the optic as part of the procedure. For this reason, I prefer topical 1% tropicamide and 2.5% phenylephrine because they allow for a good response to intracameral acetylcholine to constrict the pupil when needed. Even without preoperative mydriasis, intracameral lidocaine can dilate the pupil adequately early on, while still allowing it to respond to acetylcholine.

The simplest form of decentered sulcus IOL management is manipulation, with reorientation of the haptics into meridians where capsule and zonule support appears adequate. I consider this a viable option when there is at least 270 degrees of contiguous support. A combination of Sinskey and Kuglen hooks placed through the paracentesis tracts are used within viscoelastic to rotate the optic and haptics. There is always a tendency for the IOL to rotate back to the meridian lacking sulcus support and eventually decenter again. In these seemingly simple cases, I like to place a single peripheral McCannel suture to fixate one haptic to the iris to prevent rotation and secure the desired orientation. This is somewhat analogous to the effect of a steering-wheel lock.

The majority of freely mobile out-of-the-bag IOLs are best managed with peripheral iris suture fixation of the haptics using a modified McCannel approach, with some form of Siepser sliding knots.[2,3] I begin with mild pharmacologic dilation, followed by topical tetracaine and intracameral 1.5% preservative-free lidocaine for anesthesia. A nonretentive viscoelastic is used to stabilize anterior chamber depth and encase the IOL for support during manipulation. I am careful not to overinflate the chamber to best achieve a planar iris contour. I then bring the optic anterior to the pupil, with either hooks or a microforceps, and attempt to capture it with the pupil. I often will add the acetylcholine with one hand through the side port, while supporting the IOL with the other hand. Capturing the optic by the pupil is the key maneuver. It generally is manageable with any 3-piece IOL and reasonable pupil anatomy (Figure 48-2). Following optic capture, the addition of viscoelastic over the iris in the region of the peripheral haptics easily will delineate the actual haptic location and facilitate accurate suture passage. At this point, I select an appropriate limbal paracentesis site to introduce the suture. I find it works best to create the entry paracentesis for the needle approximately 1 to 2 clock-hours away from the actual peripheral haptic location. The paracentesis should be just inside the limbus and oriented fairly tangential to it. These factors allow good visualization of the needle tip as it is passed through the iris and avoidance of an overly steep needle angle. After the needle is passed through the peripheral iris and behind the haptic, simply lifting the needle slightly should create movement of the entire IOL, confirming that I will have the haptic included in the suture bite. I bring the needle tip up through the iris and directly out through any nearby area of clear cornea (Figure 48-3). Although the 2 suture ends can be retrieved through another common paracentesis created over the haptic to complete a knot, I find a Siepser sliding-knot technique provides more precise knot tensioning and better security.[4]

The Siepser sliding knot can be achieved by starting with the suture passed through a paracentesis, under the IOL haptic, and out the clear cornea (Figure 48-4). The distal intraocular segment of the suture is retrieved with a Kuglen hook, or similar instrument, and externalized back out the entry paracentesis (Figure 48-5). This will create a loop of suture that will be used to tie the Siepser sliding knot. Before tying the suture, it is important to identify the portion of the retrieved

Figure 48-2. (A) A combination of hooks is used to bring the optic above the iris plane for capture. (B) Capture is completed with the addition of acetylcholine to induce miosis.

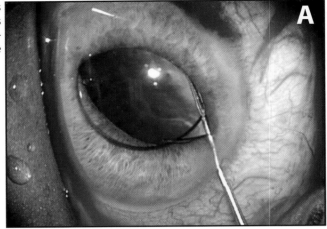

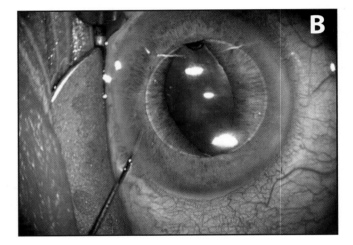

loop that comes from the distal iris, rather than from the distal cornea. The 2 externalized suture ends then are grasped with forceps, and a double throw is tied (Figures 48-6 and 48-7). The trailing suture segment is then stabilized and gentle traction is placed on the distal suture segment as the knot is gathered and pulled into the anterior chamber to secure the haptic (see Figure 48-7). Finally, the suture ends are cut short with intraocular scissors. The second haptic is fixed in this same manner and the optic is prolapsed back into the posterior chamber.

I consider repairing a deformed pupil either prior to attempting optic capture or at the conclusion of the IOL fixation. In cases associated with moderate traumatic mydriasis, I prefer pupilloplasty as an initial step to improve subsequent capture of the IOL optic. Any vitreous prolapse must be managed using proper vitrectomy instrumentation. I use the handpiece without an irrigating sleeve and obtain inflow via an anterior chamber–maintaining cannula.

Unlike a 3-piece IOL, achieving temporary optic capture of a large, single-piece PMMA IOL often is more challenging because the large diameter and more rigid haptics tend to keep the entire lens trapped posterior to the ciliary body. This can create severe posterior vaulting away from the pupil plane. I usually consider ab-externo scleral fixation for these cases. I create a conjunctiva peritomy at the site of a desired fixation point, and a midperipheral cornea paracentesis is made 180 degrees away. A hollow 26-gauge needle is placed through the sclera at the desired fixation

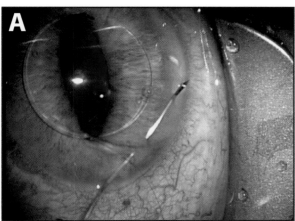

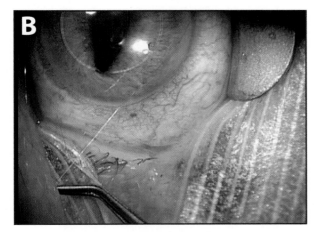

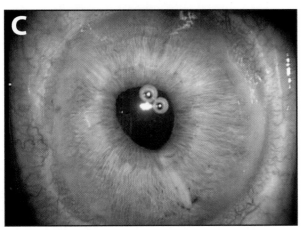

Figure 48-3. (A) The needle has been passed through the paracentesis, through the iris, behind the haptic, back out through the iris and through an area of distal clear cornea. (B) A Siepser sliding knot is preferred in this case to secure the haptics to the peripheral iris. (C) After the haptics are secured, the optic is prolapsed back into the posterior chamber, and the sutures are barely visible in the periphery at the 5-o'clock and 10-o'clock positions.

site within a shallow scleral groove 1.5 mm behind the limbus. The tip of the needle is brought into the pupillary zone. One end of a double-armed, 9-0 polypropylene suture on a long needle is passed through the clear corneal paracentesis and into the tip of the hollow 26-gauge needle. Both of these are withdrawn externally from the sclera. The 26-gauge needle is placed again through

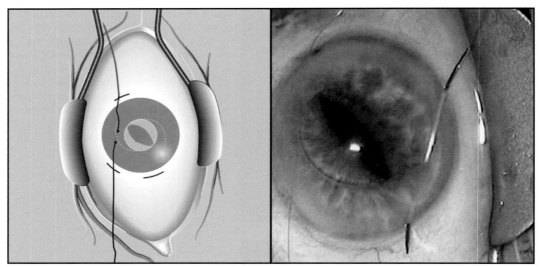

Figure 48-4. Properly placed suture under the IOL haptic.

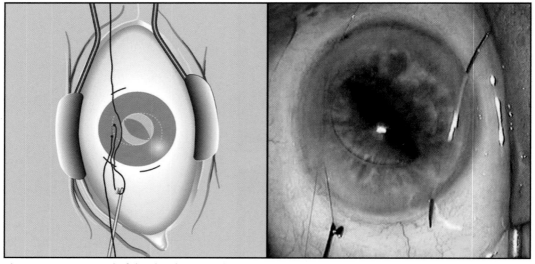

Figure 48-5. Retrieval of the distal intraocular suture segment through the paracentesis.

the scleral fixation site 1 mm away from the first pass. At this time, an iris spatula or hook can be used to elevate the malpositioned IOL up to the iris plane. The tip of the hollow needle is passed beneath the free-floating haptic and then above the optic to meet with the other end of the polypropylene suture that has been placed through the same corneal paracentesis as the first. This needle is brought out through the sclera as tension is applied to the other side of the suture to secure the haptic. The suture knot is rotated into the sclera. Visualization can be improved dramatically with the placement of 2 nylon iris retractors through the peripheral clear cornea in the region of refixation.

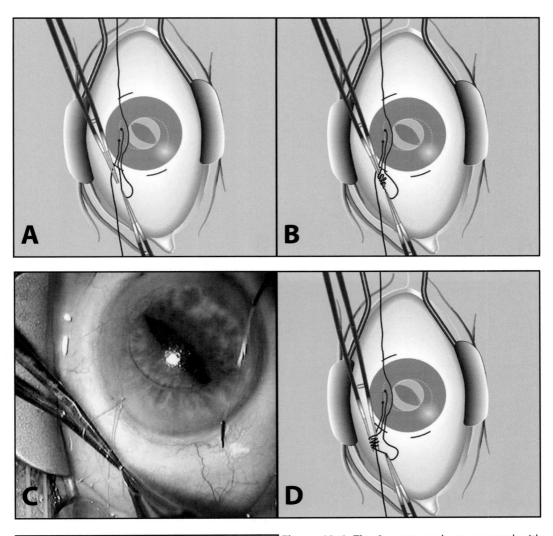

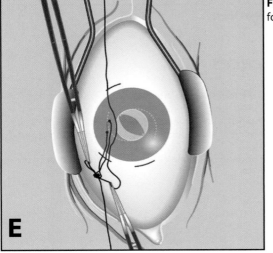

Figure 48-6. The 2 suture ends are grasped with forceps and a double throw is tied.

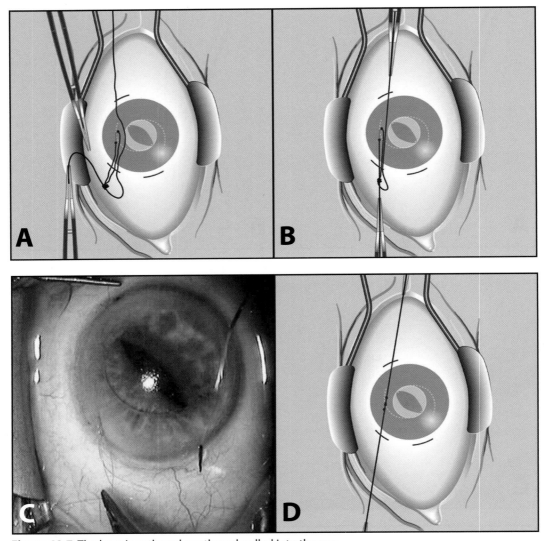

Figure 48-7. The knot is gathered gently and pulled into the eye.

References

1. Masket S, Osher RH. Late complications with intraocular lens dislocation after capsulorrhexis in pseudoexfoliation syndrome. *J Cataract Refract Surg.* 2002;28(8):1481-1484.
2. Siepser SB. The closed chamber slipping suture technique for iris repair. *Ann Ophthalmol.* 1994;26(3):71-72.
3. Chang DF. Siepser slipknot for McCannel iris-suture fixation of subluxated intraocular lenses. *J Cataract Refract Surg.* 2004;30(6):1170-1176.
4. Condon GP. Peripheral iris fixation of a foldable acrylic posterior chamber intraocular lens in the absence of capsule support. *Techniques in Ophthalmology.* 2004;2:104-109.

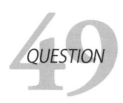
MY PSEUDOEXFOLIATION PATIENT HAS NEWLY DISCOVERED PSEUDOPHACODONESIS 5 YEARS FOLLOWING SURGERY. HOW SHOULD I PROCEED?

Alan S. Crandall, MD

Pseudoexfoliation syndrome, found in up to 35% of patients 70 years and older, is a relatively common systemic disorder with well-known ocular sequelae.[1] A deposition of an ancillary fibrillary substance is on all structures of the anterior chamber (Figure 49-1). Of course, pseudoexfoliation is highly associated with glaucoma and with complications during cataract extractions.[2,3] The iris involvement may lead to poor pupil dilation, which further increases the risk for cataract surgery complications. The accumulation of pseudoexfoliation material is associated with a proteolytic process that probably leads to decreased tensile strength in the zonules.[4] The capsule is also more brittle in pseudoexfoliation syndrome. Fortunately, with modern phacoemulsification techniques, such as continuous curvilinear capsulorrhexis, chopping, and the use of capsular tension rings (CTRs) or capsule retractors, the surgical complication rate in these eyes has dropped dramatically.[5]

Dislocation of Intraocular Lens and Bag Complex

Late spontaneous dislocation of the entire intraocular lens (IOL) and bag complex in pseudoexfoliation also has been reported (Figure 49-2).[6,7] The dislocation may occur 2 months to 17 years postoperatively, and the average is approximately 8.5 years after surgery.[8] Pseudoexfoliation has been significantly associated with late IOL dislocations.

Most patients do not present to the ophthalmologist until the entire bag–IOL complex has completely dislocated. However, some patients may note fluctuating vision and may present with pseudophacodonesis and minimal subluxation. Surgical management is certainly easier the sooner the patient presents.

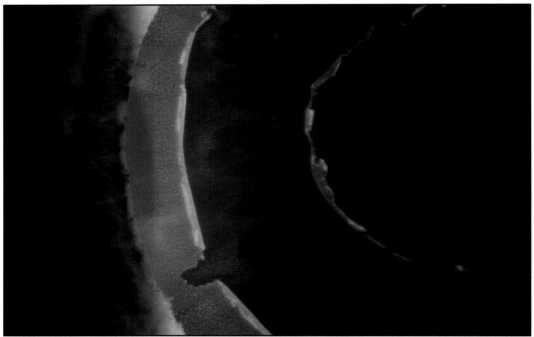

Figure 49-1. Pseudoexfoliation material seen on the anterior capsule.

SURGICAL MANAGEMENT

Surgical management of the bag–IOL dislocation depends on the type of IOL. For silicone plate haptic IOLs, there is no other choice than to explant the bag–IOL complex and, following an anterior vitrectomy, replace it with an anterior chamber IOL, an iris-fixated IOL, or a sclerally fixated IOL. Intraocular lenses with loop haptics, however, can be suture fixated either to the sclera or to the iris.

Multiple techniques exist for scleral fixation; however, my preferred technique is one that was recently modified by Kirk and Condon.[9] I have found this new technique to be a simplified version of previous techniques that minimize complex manipulations. As soon as the position of the haptics is known and a decision is made where to place the sutures, a 4-to 5-mm conjunctival peritomy is made (fornix based), approximately 180 degrees apart. Two marks are made 2 mm posterior to the limbus. A 23-gauge MVR microviteoretina blade is used to make 2 entrances into the eye. It is important to direct the blade perpendicular to the sclera (toward the optic nerve) first and then parallel, but behind the iris. This is repeated 180 degrees away. A 9-0 PROLENE suture on a CTC-6 needle (Ethicon) is then passed through one site deep into the bag complex and then through (encircling the haptic or CTR, if present). The needle then is directed through the peripheral cornea and out. Through the other incision site, a hook or 25-gauge ILM forceps (Grieshaber Instrumentation, Alcon Laboratories) is placed above the bag complex, retrieving the suture and then lassoing the complex. The advantage of this technique is in the simplicity: no docking of needles is necessary, and thus, intraocular manipulations are minimized. The same process is completed at the site 180 degrees away. Sutures are tied and rotated into the scleral incision, and then the conjunctiva is closed. The vitreous stain, either Kenalog (triamcinolone) or Triescence (my preference [triamcinolone]), is injected and the anterior vitrectomy is completed.

In contrast to scleral fixation, one may fixate the haptics of the IOL to the iris. First, bring the complex up to the pupillary plane,[10] where vitreous and the surrounding capsular remnants are

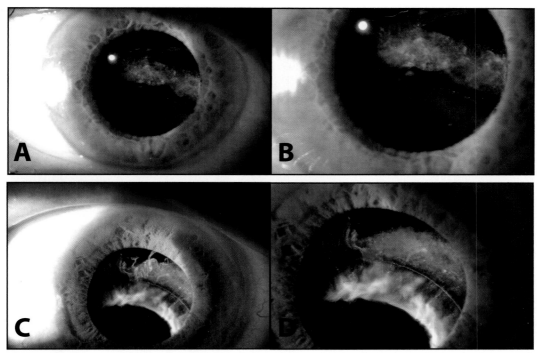

Figure 49-2. Clinical presentation of late in-the-bag dislocation of an IOL in a patient with a history of pseudoexfoliation.

removed with a vitrectomy handpiece. I then use a double-armed, 10-0 polypropylene suture to fixate each haptic to the peripheral iris with a modified McCannel suture (Figure 49-3).

As a possible preventive measure, some surgeons advocate making a relaxing cut in the capsulorrhexis margin after the IOL has been implanted. Alternatively, this can be done postoperatively with the yttrium aluminum garnet (YAG) laser.

These strategies have not been tested by a randomized study and because this is such a late postoperative complication, it will take a long time to prove whether any preventive measure is effective. Others feel that implanting a CTR may help by redistributing and resisting capsular contractile forces more evenly (Figure 49-4). Although CTRs may help to prevent capsular contraction, as bag dislocation is due to progressive zonular weakness, they probably will not stop the process. One advantage of having a CTR in the bag would be that it could be used to fixate the complex sclerally.

A final option is to use a modified CTR, such as a Cionni I or II (FCI Ophthalmics), which has an eyelet that can be used for scleral suture fixation.[8] However, HARP (high-gain avalanche rushing-amorphous photoconductor) camera views in cadaver eyes show that inserting these CTRs can cause significant iatrogenic damage to the zonules.[9,11] Because the incidence of late bag–IOL dislocation is probably low, one must carefully weigh the risks of inserting these devices against the theoretical benefit.

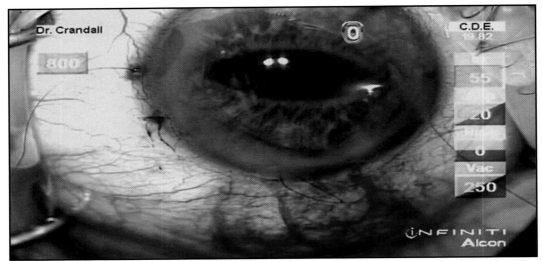

Figure 49-3. Double-armed 10-0 polypropylene suture to fixate each haptic to the peripheral iris with a modified McCannel suture.

Figure 49-4. Scleral fixation of the lens with a capsular tension ring.

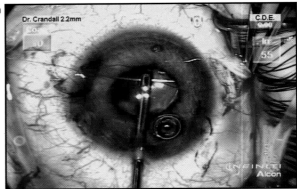

Conclusion

Late dislocation of the entire bag–IOL complex in pseudoexfoliation is unusual but not rare. Careful postoperative follow-up of pseudoexfoliation patients is important and may afford an earlier opportunity for corrective surgery (Figure 49-5). Recommendations include making a capsulorrhexis that is relatively large (5.5 mm) and promptly treating any capsular phimosis with YAG laser relaxing cuts. Whether to implant a CTR routinely in every pseudoexfoliation patient is controversial and probably is not necessary.

References

1. Naumann GO, Schlotzer-Schrehardt U, Kuchle M. Pseudoexfoliation syndrome for the comprehensive ophthalmologist. Intraocular and systemic manifestations. *Ophthalmology.* 1998;105(6):951-968.
2. Avramides S, Traianidis P, Sakkias G. Cataract surgery and lens implantation in eyes with exfoliation syndrome. *J Cataract Refract Surg.* 1997;23(4):583-587.

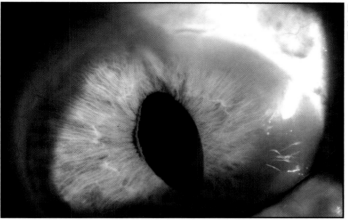

Figure 49-5. Postoperative results showing a well-centered intraocular lens.

3. Bartholomew RS. Lens displacement associated with pseudocapsular exfoliation. A report on 19 cases in the Southern Bantu. *Br J Ophthalmol.* 1970;54(11):744-750.

4. Skuta GL, Parrish RK 2nd, Hodapp E, Forster RK, Rockwood EJ. Zonular dialysis during extracapsular cataract extraction in pseudoexfoliation syndrome. *Arch Ophthalmol.* 1987;105(5):632-634.

5. Fine IH, Hoffman RS. Phacoemulsification in the presence of pseudoexfoliation: challenges and options. *J Cataract Refract Surg.* 1997;23(2):160-165.

6. Jehan FS, Mamalis N, Crandall AS. Spontaneous late dislocation of intraocular lens within the capsular bag in pseudoexfoliation patients. *Ophthalmology.* 2001;108(10):1727-1731.

7. Pueringer SL, Hodge DO, Erie JC. Risk of late intraocular lens dislocation after cataract surgery, 1980-2009: a population-based study. *Am J Ophthalmol.* 2011;152(4):618-623.

8. Davis D, Brubaker J, Espandar L, et al. Late in-the-bag spontaneous intraocular lens dislocation: evaluation of 86 consecutive cases. *Ophthalmology.* 2009;116(4):664-670.

9. Kirk TQ, Condon GP. Simplified ab externo scleral fixation for late in-the-bag intraocular lens dislocation. *J Cataract Refract Surg.* 2012;38(10):1711-1715.

10. Chang DF. Viscoelastic levitation of posteriorly dislocated intraocular lenses from the anterior vitreous. *J Cataract Refract Surg.* 2002;28(9):1515-1519.

11. Miyake K, Ota I, Miyake S, Tanioka K, Kubota M, Mochizuki R. Application of a newly developed, highly sensitive camera and a 3-dimensional high-definition television system in experimental ophthalmic surgeries. *Arch Ophthalmol.* 1999;117(12):1623-1629.

FINANCIAL DISCLOSURES

Dr. Iqbal Ike K. Ahmed has no financial or proprietary interest in the materials presented herein.

Dr. Eric C. Amesbury has no financial or proprietary interest in the materials presented herein.

Dr. Lisa Brothers Arbisser is on the Optimedica Surgeons' council and had an honorarium from Bausch & Lomb Inc this year.

Dr. Rosa Braga-Mele has no financial or proprietary interest in the materials presented herein.

Dr. David F. Chang is a consultant for Abbott Medical Optics Inc.

Dr. Steve Charles is a consultant for Alcon Laboratories and Topcon Medical Laser Systems.

Dr. Theodore J. Christakis has no financial or proprietary interest in the materials presented herein.

Dr. Fred Chu has no financial or proprietary interest in the materials presented herein.

Dr. Robert J. Cionni is a consultant for Alcon Laboratories.

Dr. Garry P. Condon is a consultant and is on the speakers bureau for Alcon Laboratories, Allergan Inc, and MicroSurgical Technology.

Dr. Alan S. Crandall is a consultant for Alcon Laboratories, AqueSys Inc, Ivantis Inc, and Omeros.

Dr. Mahshad Darvish has no financial or proprietary interest in the materials presented herein.

Dr. Derek W. DelMonte has no financial or proprietary interest in the materials presented herein.

Dr. Uday Devgan has no financial or proprietary interest in the materials presented herein.

Dr. Dipanjal Dey has no financial or proprietary interest in the materials presented herein.

Dr. Deepinder K. Dhaliwal has no financial or proprietary interest in the materials presented herein.

Dr. Paul Ernest has no financial or proprietary interest in the materials presented herein.

Dr. William J. Fishkind is a consultant for Abbott Medical Optics Inc and LensAR Inc and has financial interest in Thieme Publishers Royalty.

Dr. Nicole R. Fram is a lecturer for Alcon Laboratories and Bausch & Lomb Inc and has received a grant from Accutome Inc.

Dr. Scott Greenbaum has no financial or proprietary interest in the materials presented herein.

Dr. Preeya K. Gupta has no financial or proprietary interest in the materials presented herein.

Dr. David R. Hardten has been a consultant for Abbott Medical Optics Inc.

Dr. Mojgan Hassanlou has no financial or proprietary interest in the materials presented herein.

Dr. Bonnie An Henderson has no financial or proprietary interest in the materials presented herein.

Dr. Warren E. Hill is a consultant for Alcon Laboratories.

Dr. Richard S. Hoffman has no financial or proprietary interest in the materials presented herein.

Dr. Edward Holland is a consultant for Abbott Medical Optics Inc, Alcon Laboratories, Bausch & Lomb Inc, Senju Pharmaceutical Co, WaveTec Vision, SARCode Bioscience Inc, and TearScience; receives grant support from Abbott Medical Optics Inc, Alcon Laboratories, and Wavetec Vision; and receives lecture fees from Alcon Laboratories and Bausch & Lomb Inc.

Dr. Sumitra Khandelwal has no financial or proprietary interest in the materials presented herein.

Dr. Terry Kim has no financial or proprietary interest in the materials presented herein.

Dr. Gaston O. Lacayo III has no financial or proprietary interest in the materials presented herein.

Dr. Stephen S. Lane is a consultant for Alcon Laboratories, Bausch & Lomb Inc, Abbott Medical Optics Inc, ISTA Pharmaceuticals Inc, PowerVision Inc, VisionCare Inc, WaveTec Vision, SARCode Bioscience Inc, Pharmaceutical Research Network, and TearScience.

Dr. Richard A. Lewis is a consultant for Aerie Pharmaceuticals Inc, Alcon Laboratories, Allergan Inc, AqueSys Inc, Advanced Vision Science Inc, Ivantis Inc, and Merck.

Dr. Richard L. Lindstrom has financial interest in Alcon Laboratories, Abbott Medical Optics Inc, and Bausch & Lomb Inc.

Dr. Brian Little has no financial or proprietary interest in the materials presented herein.

Dr. Francis S. Mah has financial interest in Alcon Laboratories, Allergan Inc, Bausch & Lomb Inc.

Dr. Parag Majmudar is a consultant for Bausch & Lomb Inc, Allergan Inc, Alcon Laboratories, and TearScience.

Dr. Boris Malyugin has financial interest in the Malyugin Ring pupil expansion device.

Dr. Nick Mamalis is an editor for the *Journal of Cataract and Refractive Surgery*.

Dr. Samuel Masket is a consultant for Alcon Laboratories, Haag-Streit, Ocular Therapeutix Inc, PowerVision Inc, and WaveTec Vision; is a lecturer for Alcon Laboratories, Bausch & Lomb Inc, and Carl Zeiss Meditec Inc; and received a grant from Accutome Inc.

Dr. Kevin M. Miller has no financial or proprietary interest in the materials presented herein.

Dr. Christina S. Moon has no financial or proprietary interest in the materials presented herein.

Dr. Kristiana D. Neff has no financial or proprietary interest in the materials presented herein.

Dr. Louis D. "Skip" Nichamin is a medical monitor for Bausch & Lomb Inc. He has no financial interest in any instrument that bears his name.

Dr. Thomas A. Oetting has no financial or proprietary interest in the materials presented herein.

Dr. Randall J. Olson has no financial or proprietary interest in the materials presented herein.

Dr. Robert H. Osher is a consultant for Alcon Laboratories, Advanced Medical Optics Inc, Bausch & Lomb Inc, and Carl Zeiss Meditec Inc.

Dr. Mark Packer has no financial or proprietary interest in the materials presented herein.

Dr. Mauricio A. Perez has no financial or proprietary interest in the materials presented herein.

Dr. Michael B. Raizman is a consultant for Alcon Laboratories, Allergan Inc, and Bausch & Lomb Inc.

Dr. Thomas Samuelson is a consultant for Alcon Laboratories, AcuMEMS Inc, Allergan Inc, Abbott Medical Optics Inc, AqueSys Inc, Endo Optiks, Glaukos Corporation, Ivantis Inc, Merck, *Ocular Surgery News*, QLT Inc, Santen Pharmaceutical Co., Ltd., and SLACK Incorporated.

Dr. Barry Seibel receives royalty from SLACK Incorporated.

Dr. Eric J. Sigler has no financial or proprietary interest in the materials presented herein.

Dr. Michael E. Snyder is a consultant for Alcon Laboratories, Haag-Streit, HumanOptics, and MicroSurgical Technology and a researcher for Alcon Laboratories, Haag-Streit, HumanOptics, and Ocular Therapeutix Inc.

Dr. Roger F. Steinert is a consultant and medical monitor for Abbott Medical Optics Inc.

Dr. Geoffery C. Tabin has no financial or proprietary interest in the materials presented herein.

Dr. Benjamin Thomas has no financial or proprietary interest in the materials presented herein.

Dr. Richard Tipperman is a consultant for Alcon Laboratories.

Dr. William Trattler is a consultant for Bausch & Lomb Inc, Allergan Inc, LensAR Inc, and Abbott Medical Optics Inc; receives funding for research from Bausch & Lomb Inc, Allergan Inc, and Abbott Medical Optics Inc; and receives speaker fees from Bausch & Lomb Inc, Allergan Inc, Oculus Inc, and LensAR Inc.

Dr. Farrell C. Tyson has not disclosed any relevant financial relationships.

Dr. Robin R. Vann is on the Alcon Speaker's bureau and receives honoraria for speaking on refractive cataract surgery, biometry, and IOL calculations.

Dr. David T. Vroman has no financial or proprietary interest in the materials presented herein.

Dr. R. Bruce Wallace III is a consultant for LensAR Inc and Bausch & Lomb Inc.

Dr. Keith A. Warren has no financial or proprietary interest in the materials presented herein.

Dr. Sonia H. Yoo is a consultant for Alcon Laboratories, Bausch & Lomb Inc, Optimedica, and Transcend Medical Inc, and receives grant support from Alcon Laboratories, Allergan Inc, and Carl Zeiss Meditec Inc and lecture fees from SLACK Incorporated.

INDEX